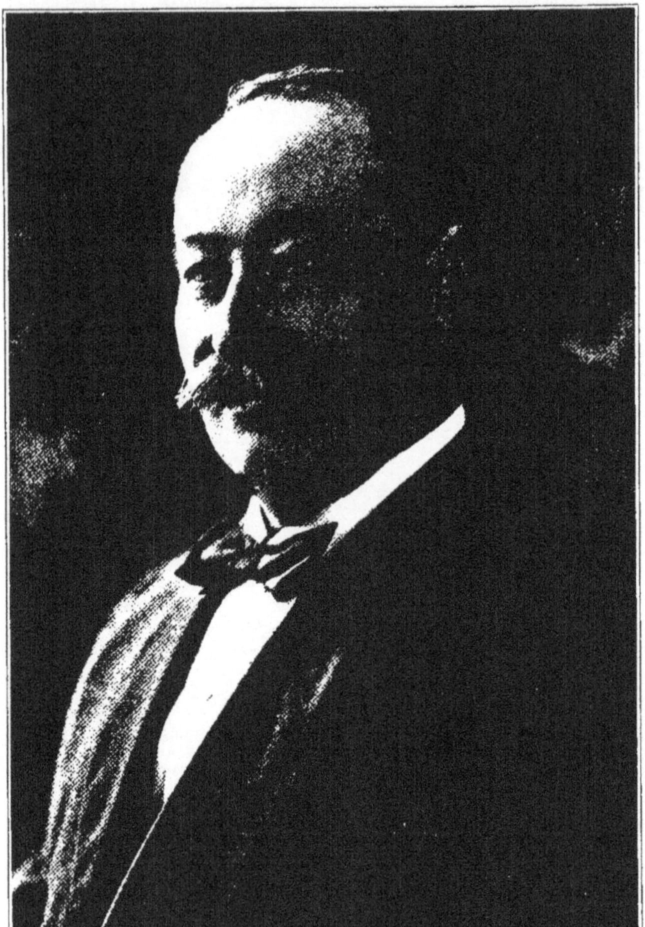

FRANK KLEINHEINZ

Completed 30 years of service in charge of the University of Wisconsin Flocks, April 8, 1920.

SHEEP MANAGEMENT
BREEDS AND JUDGING

A TEXTBOOK

FOR THE

SHEPHERD AND STUDENT

BY

FRANK KLEINHEINZ

ASSISTANT PROFESSOR OF ANIMAL HUSBANDRY
UNIVERSITY OF WISCONSIN

FIFTH EDITION

Published by the Author
MADISON, WISCONSIN
1920

Cantwell Printing Company
Madison, Wisconsin

PREFACE

There are several books on sheep husbandry written by good authorities on the subject which have been of great aid to flockmasters. However, there is need for a book written in simple, comprehensible, every-day language dealing with the practical problems of sheep husbandry. This book has been prepared not only to serve the shepherd in his every-day work, but also to meet the requirements of the student in the classroom.

Numerous inquiries from flockowners from many sections of the country for information relative to sheep husbandry and the troubles connected with the industry, the requests of many friends and students, and especially the urgent requests of Dean Henry and later of Dean Russell, both of the College of Agriculture of the University of Wisconsin, have induced the author to prepare this book. Judging from many letters received, not only the beginners with sheep, but also some of the more experienced men, often have many difficulties.

In addition to the chapters on the care and management of the flock, illustrations showing a practical method of judging sheep, together with descriptions and the scale of points of the different breeds of sheep are given.

In this work the author has given his many years experience in sheep husbandry. From his early boyhood in his native land of Bavaria, Germany, he was in charge of the flock of Shropshires on his father's farm. In America he has had charge of the flock of the Agricultural Experiment Station of the University of Wisconsin ever since April, 1890. While at this Station, he has carried on many experiments with sheep which have furnished him with a fund of valuable information regarding many lines of sheep husbandry. From all this experience, the writer feels free to state that no one man knows everything concerning sheep. Entirely new problems occasionally arise which must be solved. However, one fact is always true. This is that good judgment, energy, kindness, and painstaking care are the keynotes to success in sheep husbandry. No person who treats his sheep like scavengers, giving them little or no attention, not furnishing them half enough to eat, and even depriving them of a drink of fresh water, can ever expect to derive any pleasure or profit from sheep husbandry. For such a man the sheep will never prove to be the "Golden Hoof." No rough, brutal person possessing a violent temper and lacking self-control should ever undertake to raise or care for a flock, as such actions are entirely foreign to the innocent, peaceful nature of the sheep.

The writer feels deeply indebted to Messrs. F. B. Morrison, J. C. Marquis, and W. A. Sumner for their assistance in the preparation of this work, and also to the American Sheep Breeder for furnishing some of the photographs of prize winners.

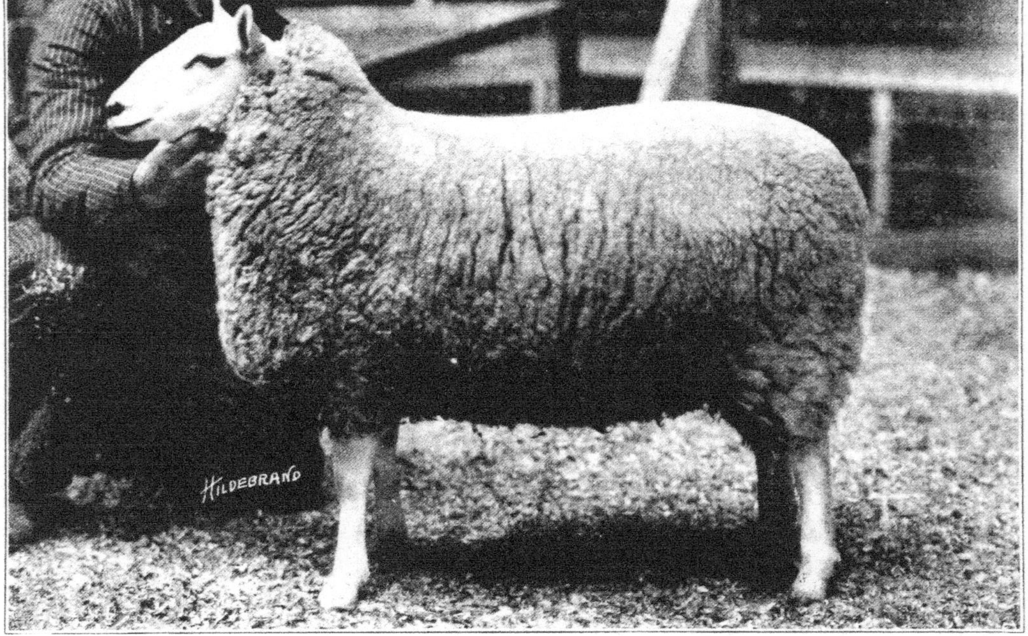

First prize and champion Cheviot ewe lamb at the International, 1917, shown by the University of Wisconsin.

CONTENTS

CHAPTER IV.

Rearing the Lambs.

CHAPTER V.

Shearing and Dipping the Flock.

CHAPTER VI.

Prevention and Treatment of Parasites.

CHAPTER VII.

Summer Feeding and Care.

CHAPTER VIII.

Feeding Sheep for Market.

CHAPTER IX.

Fitting Sheep for the Show Ring.

CHAPTER X.

Fitting Wethers for Shows.

CHAPTER XI.

The Art and Method of Judging Sheep.

CHAPTER XII.

Classification of the Breeds of Sheep.

LIST OF ILLUSTRATIONS

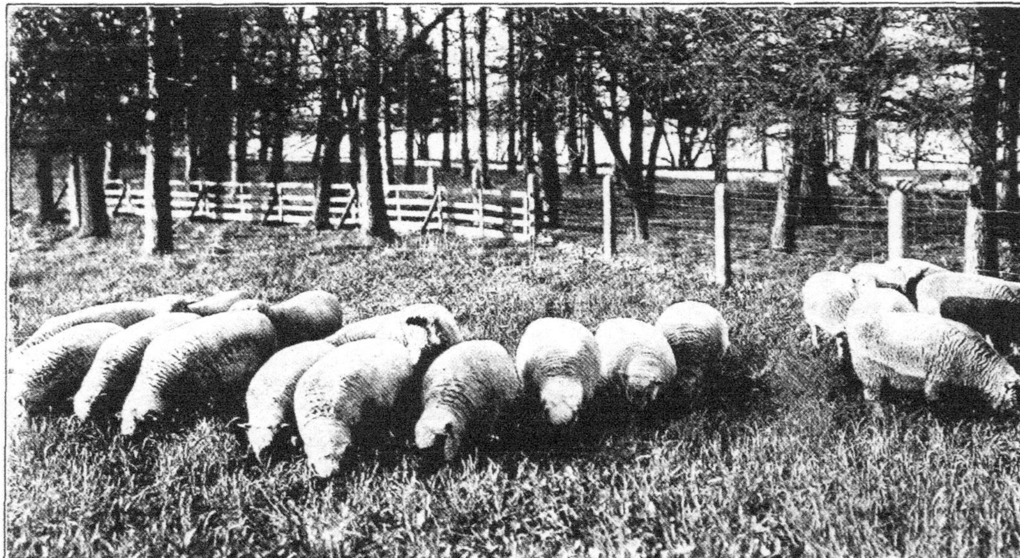

PLATE 2. A group of yearling wethers under preparation at the University of Wisconsin for the International of 1910.

INTRODUCTION

THE SHEPHERD AND HIS CALLING.

The young man with a born love for sheep is the one, as a rule, who will strive in his younger years either to find employment with some flockowner, or perhaps to engage for himself in sheep husbandry. He likes sheep, he likes to feed and take care of them. Such men, when they have learned the details connected with the business, are those who achieve the best results.

It makes no difference what breed of sheep a shepherd handles; to be successful he must practice the secrets which are the keynote to success if steadily followed, or on the other hand, which when slighted, lead to certain failure in the business. Let me mention a few of these secrets:

1. The shepherd must be kind at all times to every member of his flock.

2. He must practice cleanliness, which means to keep feed troughs clean and sweet and not let them become filthy with manure, thereby causing a disagreeable odor.

3. He must be punctual, which means to keep regular feeding hours.

4. He must use good, sound judgment in the every-day work.

5. He must feed liberally and not hold the wrong idea that sheep can live on little or nothing.

Wherever these few points are constantly observed and practiced, there need be no fear that misfortunes will come to the flock. Most of the failures in sheep husbandry may be attributed directly to carelessness and negligence on the part of the shepherd, for no breed of sheep will do well under the management of a shiftless man. A disinterested shepherd who has no interest in the welfare of his flock is just as bad as dogs that get among the flock and destroy them. Many times a shepherd does not think and does not use a little common horse sense, and then attributes everything that has gone wrong to bad luck. When we see a poor flock we generally find a poor shepherd back of it.

Many of these would be benefited if they could take a trip to England and learn from the successful flock owners of that country how they handle their flocks, and after studying their methods of raising sheep, on their way back, could go through Canada and especially through Ontario and see how our Canadian friends conduct the business. While once in a while unfavorable conditions and environment may bring about trouble, in the majority of cases the fault lies with the shepherd himself and is so often wrongly called "bad luck." If he does not care to handle his flock of breeding ewes during winter in such a manner as to assure the largest percentage of lambs, and is not willing to sit up part of the night during lambing time, he is not worth having around the flock. He must really feel proud of his success and must feel ashamed of things which have gone wrong through his fault. The best shepherds of today are not conceited over their success, but feel that there is still a little more to be learned. If a shepherd cannot at any time agree with his employer he will never take the best interest in his flock. A shepherd who walks through the sheep-fold without the necessary sharpness to detect an ill sheep in the flock is by no means the right kind of a shepherd. Another one that sees an ailing sheep, but has not energy enough to care for it at once, is just as bad or worse than the first man mentioned.

When a man does not mind the bleat of a sheep or lamb that wants more feed, salt, or water, he has not the true spirit of a shepherd. Neither is he worthy of the name of shepherd if he does not do *at once* those things which should be attended to, but says he will do them tomorrow or some other time. The man who is not aware of the danger of sheep becoming infested with maggots during hot weather and fly time, when some poor innocent sheep may be eaten alive by these pests, must certainly be a very poor shepherd or flock-master. Another who does not dip his sheep and lets ticks or lice constantly annoy and feed on them is just as cruel to his flock as the one who starves his sheep to death. If a shepherd likes to be away from his flock as much as possible he is not the one who has the thrift and welfare of it at heart; such a man had better engage in some other line of work.

Is it not good practice to go through the pasture once a day, where the sheep are grazing, to see whether a fine broad-backed ewe has not turned over on her back, with her four legs up, in a little depression in the ground, where she will die if she is not freed from this position? The shepherd who does not care about the loss of a sheep or lamb should no longer have charge of the flock. The men who do not see the importance of keeping their sheep out of cold rains and storms in late fall, winter, and early spring often have to suffer the loss of one or more members of their flock. The shepherd who has not learned the necessity of keeping the hoofs of his flock in proper trim and shape will cause much trouble in his flock and will reduce his profits. If he is not careful to avoid feeding moldy and spoiled feed of any kind to his flock, he is not a true shepherd; neither is the man who feeds frozen roots or frozen corn silage, both of which often prove fatal. Whoever believes that the best results can be obtained by merely looking at a flock, and does not go to work, is badly mistaken.

If the shepherd does not supply his flock with fresh, pure water every day in the year, but shares the opinion of quite a number of men that sheep need little or no water, he should learn as early as possible that sheep require water just as well as any other farm animal. Where the flock is allowed to drink from old stagnant water pools, the shepherd runs the risk of having his flock infested with all sorts of parasites. Failure to rub pine tar on the sheeps' noses during fly time, or to supply this in the salt trough, as is recommended elsewhere in this book, may result in the flock becoming infested with grub in the head. No flock-master can have the best results in sheep husbandry without providing some succulent feeds, such as roots, cabbage, or good, sweet corn silage, for his flock during the winter months.

The shepherd who is not aware of the serious danger of narrow doors in the sheep barn, which result in broken-down hips, pregnant ewes being induced to drop their lambs before they are due, and young lambs getting squeezed, trampled down, and killed in the rush by the older sheep, and who does nothing to prevent this evil, lacks good judgment, and is responsible for any loss incurred in this way. If a shepherd fits sheep and goes into the show ring simply to be there among the other shepherds to keep them company, and if he is not possessed with the strongest desire to win the best prizes offered, he had better stay at home and save money for his employer.

To make a long story short, a good faithful shepherd looks to every detail of his work, and has his mind, heart, and soul with his flock at all times. He leaves nothing undone which promotes the thrift and welfare of each individual sheep. He likes to talk with other successful shepherds about sheep and tries to learn the better methods. He is loyal to his employer, and works for his best interest and largest profit. His happiest hours are spent among his flock, watching young lambs grow and old ones do well. Some of the greatest men in the Old Testament were true, faithful shepherds.

Shepherd's Guide

Careful flockmasters follow these simple rules and practices to insure healthy and profitable flocks.

1. Cull the flock, sell all broken-mouthed ewes, and any other ewes that have not proved good producers.

2. Get the ewe flock in good condition before breeding begins. This insures more twins.

3. To make service easy tag all ewes before turning in ram.

4. Use a good, vigorous, pure-bred ram and do not breed more than 50 ewes to him in a season.

5. Do not use a ram lamb for breeding unless circumstances necessitate and he is unusually well-developed. If used he should not serve more than 8 to 12 ewes. Never breed ewe lambs.

6. Remove ram from flock as soon as the breeding season is over.

Shepherd's Guide—*Continued*

7. Exercise pregnant ewes as much as possible. Keep them well-sheltered, however, in wet or stormy weather.

8. Do not feed timothy or marsh hay. Clover or alfalfa are best (feed all that the flock will eat without waste). Feed corn silage or roots, 2 to 2½ pounds a head daily, to supply succulence.

9. Do not feed mouldy or frozen silage or spoiled roots to sheep. It will cause much trouble and often kill the sheep.

10. Feed some grain at least a month before lambing, ½ pound of a mixture of equal parts of oats and bran a head daily is very helpful.

11. Give close attention to the ewes at lambing time. It will save many lambs, and occasionally a mother which otherwise might die, if no help is given.

12. Pen ewe and new born lambs away from flock for a few days to prevent her from disowning them.

Shepherd's Guide—*Continued*

13. Increase the succulent feed and the grain for ewes the third day after lambing.

14. Castrate ram lambs on a bright day when one to two weeks old. Dock all lambs about a week later. Docking pinchers are recommended.

15. Wean the lambs at 4½ to 5 months of age and do not let them wean themselves. Retain all best ewe lambs for the future flock.

16. Shear the flock just as soon as the weather is warm enough to cause them to suffer from the heat. Use paper twine for tying wool.

17. Dip the whole flock about 10 days after shearing. This is very essential. Any of the standard dips may be used.

18. Feed the flock liberally.

19. Avoid parasites by changing pastures frequently. Do not allow sheep to drink stagnant water.

Shepherd's Guide—*Continued*

20. Be on the lookout for maggots in hot weather and fly-time.

21. Provide a patch of Dwarf Essex rape to furnish feed when pastures are short.

22. Good woven wire fences are necessary. Dogproof corrals safeguard sheep at night.

23. Never keep sheep on low marshy or very sandy land.

24. Provide shade for the flock in summer.

25. Supply the flock with fresh water and salt at all times. Give attention to all details and success is assured.

(Refer to index to find a more complete discussion of these subjects.)

CHAPTER I.

ESTABLISHING THE FLOCK.

THE VALUE OF SHEEP ON THE FARM.

It is generally known that, when properly managed, sheep are most profitable animals on the farm. They do not require nearly so much labor as other farm animals, especially in the summer, when the farmer is the busiest, cultivating, haying, and harvesting. Another advantage is that no expensive building is necessary for properly sheltering and housing them. Likewise the outlay of capital needed to start a flock of sheep is small compared with that required for other stock. With good prices for wool, a breeding ewe will pay for her maintenance during the year with her fleece, and will raise one or two lambs, or perhaps even three, which are net profit to the owner. With the steadily increasing demand for good mutton and the good prices paid for the same, it can easily be seen that sheep husbandry pays well, if handled in the right way.

Sheep are economical producers, and require less feed for the production of a pound of gain than the average for other classes of live stock. They have no equals as weed destroyers, for they eat nearly all of the numerous weeds and grasses which grow on the farm. The manure from sheep is worth much more per ton as fertilizer than that of any other class of farm animals except poultry. Moreover, when on pasture, sheep spread their manure more evenly than other stock. Indeed, no spreader has as yet been invented that does such perfect work as the sheep themselves. These animals never impoverish the land upon which they tread, but on the contrary build it up and improve it. For this reason the sheep is called the "Golden Hoof."

In pointing out the advantages of sheep husbandry it is not the writer's intention to urge farmers to give up all other classes of farm animals and stock up with sheep, but he wishes simply to emphasize the idea that at least a few sheep can very profitably be kept on almost all farms which are located on dry land. Sheep, however, will not thrive on marshy land.

A SMALL FLOCK FOR BEGINNERS.

It would not be wise for anyone not thoroughly familiar with sheep husbandry to start in with a large flock, for many troubles and obstacles arise which have to be overcome, and the remedies must be learned by practical experience, as all of them cannot be found in books. Many people who started in the business too heavily have made a failure of it, and consequently have been compelled to drop the undertaking. The proper procedure is to start in with a small flock and gradually increase the number, as one's knowledge of the care and management of sheep enlarges.

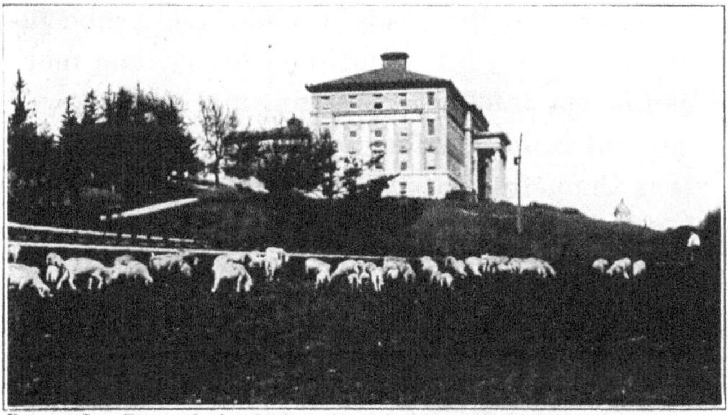

PLATE 3. Part of the University of Wisconsin flock on the campus near Agricultural Hall, right after shearing.

One of the greatest drawbacks to sheep husbandry in many sections of the country at the present time is the dog problem. It is to be hoped, however, that in every state of our country laws will be enacted similar to the laws of some states, which will do away with many of the worthless mongrel curs that cause enormous damage by killing sheep, and have frightened many small flockowners out of the business.

THE SCRUB RAM UNPROFITABLE.

Flockmasters should avoid the practice of using the grade or scrub ram, for wherever such a ram is used no improvement in the offspring can be expected. Indeed, in many cases the vitality, conformation, and strength of a flock is reduced by using an inferior grade or scrub ram for breeding. Therefore, the scrub ram, like the scrub stallion, must be driven out of the country, and more scientific and intelligent breeding must be followed if present conditions are to be improved.

It is shameful that there are so many flocks of inferior breeding and quality throughout nearly all parts of our country. Flocks of this type demand more feed and care than flocks of good breeding. Moreover, does not rearing good stock afford the farmer much greater pleasure and more encouragement than raising the inferior class commonly called "scrubs"? Does he not also know that high grade animals will return far greater profit than scrubs? The writer has spent many of the happiest hours in his life in taking care of high class animals, but he would have found no pleasure in caring for inferior ones.

It is thus evident that flockmasters should in all cases use a pure-bred ram. Not every one of these, however, is a good individual, although he may have a pedigree to his credit. Some registered rams are very inferior in type and conformation, and will not make any improvement in a flock. Breeders would improve the sheep industry if they would use the knife, and castrate all inferior buck lambs and sell them for mutton, as such rams do not uplift sheep breeding, but on the other hand degrade it.

THE SELECTION OF THE RAM.

It has been demonstrated that the ram is half, or as some breeders say, even more than half of the flock. The writer fully agrees with this statement, as he has often observed surprisingly good results from using a first-class sire on the most common kind of females. It is doubtful whether in any other line of animal breeding such rapid improvement can be accomplished by the use of good sires as in the case of sheep breeding. The best sires are none too good.

The first illustration in Plate 4 shows four Montana ewes bought on the range some years ago for $2.25 per head. These ewes were very thin when purchased and were just "sheep," for they showed no evidence of belonging to any particular breed. By the use of the pure-bred Southdown ram, which is shown in Plate 5, the seven fine, well-built lambs were raised in one season from the four ewes. One of these lambs was good enough to win the second prize at the International in a class

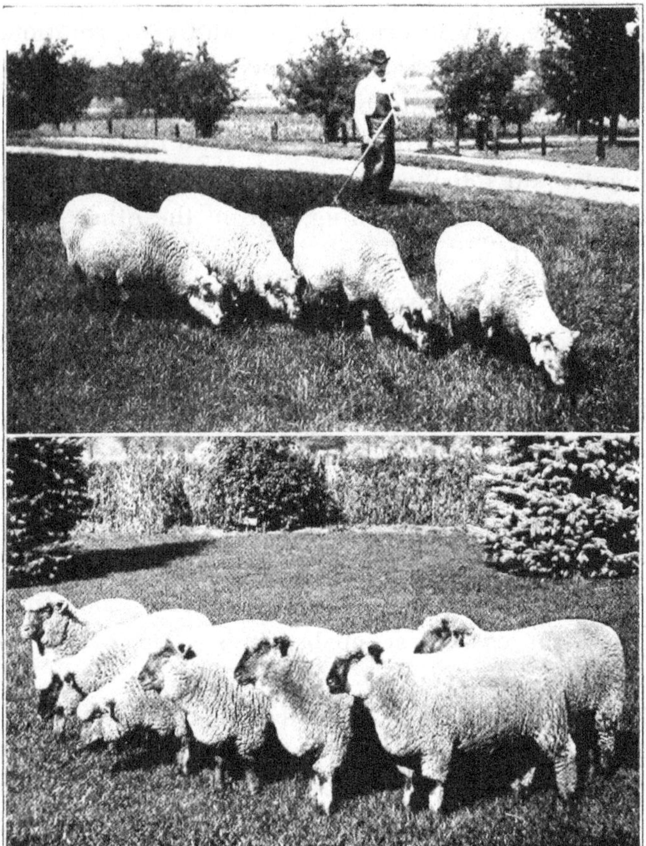

PLATE 4. (a) Four Montana ewes bought on the range for $2.25 per head. (b) Seven lambs raised from these ewes in one season. Their sire was a pure-bred.

where 38 lambs were shown. These lambs show in a striking manner what great improvement can be made by the use of a good sire on the most inferior females.

When selecting a breeding ram of a mutton breed, one should know and bear in mind the ideal of a well-built ram, possessing the right type, so as to be able at once to distinguish the good ram from the inferior one. The points of a good ram are as follows: He should possess lots of vigor and vitality, which is indicated by a short, broad head, large nostrils, bold eyes, breadth on the poll or top of the head, a short, thick neck, a wide and deep chest, broad, level shoulders—smooth on top, and a well-developed forearm. His forelegs should be straight and short, and set well apart. He should be broad and deep in the heart girth, which insures good constitution. A broad, straight back, with well-sprung ribs, is very essential. A smooth, wide, and thick loin adds greatly to the value of a sire. He should also have a long, level, and wide rump, with a full, deep twist. His hind legs, like his forelegs, should be short, straight, and wide apart, and the flank should be thick and low, forming a straight side line as well as a straight underline. The skin should be of a pink color, and the fleece long, fine, and dense, depending, of course, upon the particular breed to which he belongs.

Style and carriage are other strong points in a good ram. The fact that rams of nearly all the middle and long wool breeds should be free from

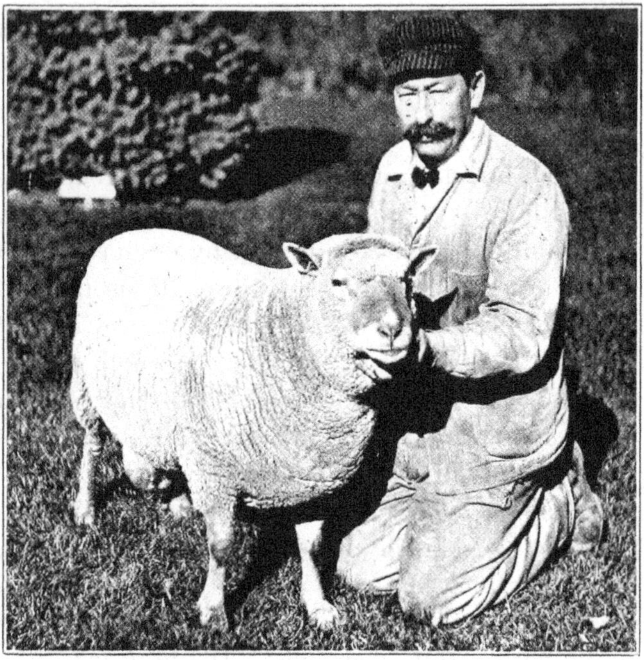

PLATE 5. Pure-bred Southdown ram. Sire of the seven lambs from Montana ewes.

horns, stubs, or scurs, should not be overlooked. Dorsets and Cheviots are exempt from this rule. The ram should show masculinity in his head and have strong bone.

Heavily fitted show rams have often failed to be breeders, or if they did breed, they produced small, weak lambs. Flockmasters are, therefore, warned not to purchase these too heavily fitted or "overdone" rams. A good, so-called "field" ram, in proper condition, generally gives the best results in breeding.

THE AGE OF THE RAM TO USE.

A ram of the middle and long wool breeds is sufficiently developed and fit for service at the age of one and one-half years, being then called a "yearling." While it is common among breeders to buy yearling rams for service, it may be of interest to flockmasters to know that it has been found here at the Wisconsin Experiment Station, where every lamb is weighed at birth, that lambs sired by rams which were older than yearlings are heavier, on an average, than those from yearlings.

Sheep breeders very often make a mistake by using a ram lamb for breeding. Such a practice is detrimental to their own interests and profit. A sheep makes its most growth the first year of its life; and hence it can readily be seen that when a lamb, only about six to eight months old, is bred to a lot of ewes, its own development is very much hindered. Ram lambs, when heavily used, have often proved to be non-breeders afterwards.

Therefore, the up-to-date sheep breeder never uses ram lambs for breeding, or at least only in rare cases. For instance, a breeder buys an exceedingly good ram lamb for a high price, which he intends to use as a yearling in his flock, and he may be very anxious to see the offspring from it. In such a case, it might be allowable to breed this ram lamb to three or perhaps even five ewes, but, of course, it would be better if the lamb is not used at all. The reason why so many ram lambs are used for breeding is that farmers can purchase a lamb a little cheaper than a yearling, but the few extra dollars saved in the purchase price are doubly lost at the other end. In the writer's opinion it is far better to buy a yearling ram instead of a lamb, because the yearling has nearly reached full development and with proper care will not change his form. In the case of the lamb, however, its future development cannot in all cases be correctly predicted, as lambs often change markedly in conformation. Indeed, the best of lambs have often turned out to be poor yearlings.

THE CARE OF THE RAM IN SUMMER.

To let the ram run with the flock during the summer and fall is not the best practice. The ram is more or less restless when in company with breeding ewes, and ewes often become pregnant and give birth to lambs at times when it is not desirable to have them come. It is a much better plan to keep the ram isolated from the flock. He can be turned into a paddock or small field where he will find enough grass to keep him in good condition. It is important that the ram have shade and fresh water where he is kept in summer, and salt is also another requisite for him. Towards fall when the weather gets colder and chilling rains frequently make it unpleasant, the ram should be housed during the night at least, for many valuable breeding rams have become stiff and rheumatic at this season, disabling them at the time needed for service, and ruining them for life.

THE RAM IN THE FALL.

It is customary to turn the ram with the flock of ewes when breeding is to begin. Although this plan is permissible, a more satisfactory method, where time will permit, is to follow what is termed "hand coupling." In hand coupling the flock of ewes to be bred to one ram is brought each morning to an enclosure where the ram is turned with them. The shepherd watches the ram closely, and as soon as any ewe has had one service she is turned out of the enclosure, so that the ram will pay attention to other ewes in heat. It is not advisable to allow the ram to breed more than three

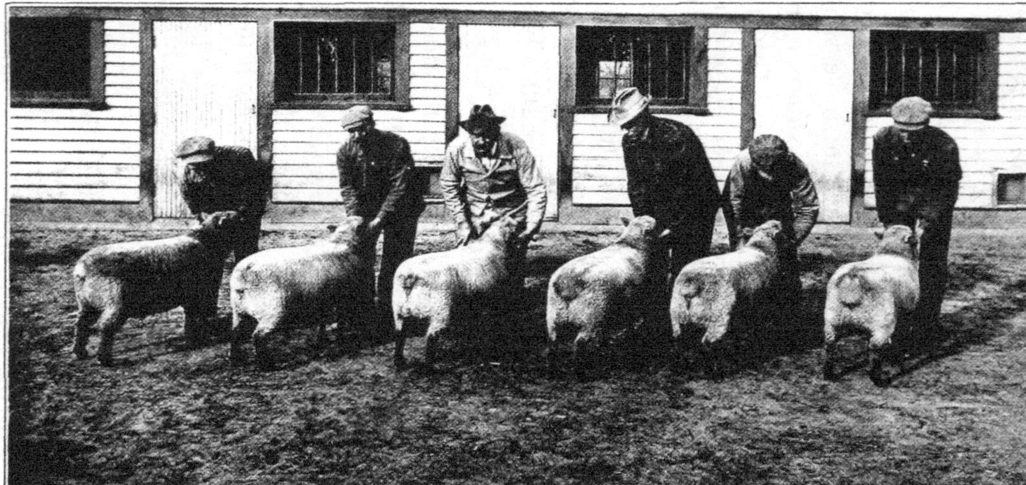

Plate 6. Purebred Southdown yearling wethers at the International, 1913. The third wether from the left was first prize and champion alive, besides being first prize and champion in the dressed carcass class. The one at the right won third prize alive, and second prize in the dressed carcass class. The third one from the right was the third prize carcass. Shown by the University of Wisconsin.

ewes in the morning. Therefore, if there should be more than three in heat in the morning the rest should be reserved for the evening.

If a ewe should fail to become pregnant from her first service, she will return in heat again in from fourteen to nineteen days. However, the great majority return in sixteen to seventeen days. Only in three or four cases has the writer known as long a period as twenty-one days to pass before ewes returned.

By the method of hand coupling the shepherd is able to keep a record of the date each ewe becomes pregnant. Hence he will know the date when she is due to lamb. When the ram is allowed to serve each ewe but once at each time she is in heat, rather than to serve her half a dozen times, his vitality and vigor are also saved to a great extent. Moreover, it is well known that a single service is better for the ewe than being bred several times.

Many sheep breeders who have not time to practice hand coupling, but nevertheless want to make sure whether the ram that is turned with the ewe flock is a breeder, paint him on the brisket between his forelegs with some color which will leave a mark of the paint on the wool of the ewe. This mark indicates that the ewe has been bred. After eighteen days or three weeks have passed,

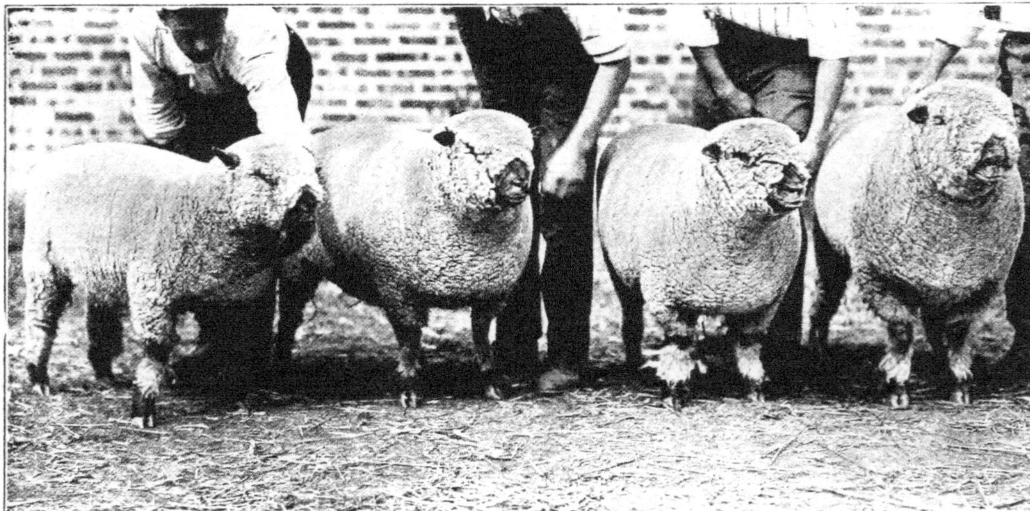

PLATE 7. Champion Shropshire flock at the International, 1910, shown by Chandler Bros.

the ram is painted with another color, and in this way the breeder is enabled to find out whether the ewes are returning or not. Some breeders put a different color on the ram the third time, and if all ewes return after being bred two or three times, another ram should be secured. The writer has seen rams that apparently did their duty well and bred many ewes, but never got a single one with lamb.

However, even if the first half dozen or so of ewes served do return, the shepherd need not necessarily worry about the ram's not being a breeder. Indeed, the writer has observed that very commonly the first few ewes bred by any ram will return.

It is a peculiar fact that where the ram is left with the flock he may pay all his attention to one ewe and entirely neglect others which are in heat, thereby needlessly wearing out his vitality. In such a case the ram seems instinctively to take a liking to this one ewe. All this will be prevented where hand coupling is followed.

THE NUMBER OF EWES ALLOWED TO ONE RAM.

Not more than fifty to fifty-five ewes should be bred to one ram in a season. The writer has observed in his many years of experience that even with this number of ewes to one ram and where hand coupling was followed, the last lambs born were not nearly as strong as those born first. This emphasizes strongly how unwise it is to allow the ram to serve too many ewes. On the western ranges where the rams run at large with the flock, and where no grain is fed them, only from thirty-five to forty ewes are allotted to each ram.

FEED FOR THE RAM.

To obtain the best results from a ram, he must be kept in a strong, vigorous condition. He needs no grain during the summer months when he has good pasture, but at least one month before breeding begins he should be given some grain. Nothing can be more highly recommended than a mixture of two parts of oats and one part of bran. This ration, which is strong in protein, does not tend to produce much fat. The amount of this mixture to be fed lies entirely in the feeder's judgment, for he must distinguish between "thrifty" and "too fat" condition. No satisfactory results can be expected from a ram that is too thin, nor from one that is too fat.

THE RAM IN WINTER.

The ram should be kept away from the breeding flock in the winter, as in summer, so that he cannot annoy and bunt the pregnant ewes around, as he may often otherwise do. If a small amount of the grain mixture, before mentioned, is given daily with some good clover or alfalfa hay, and a few roots or a little corn silage, the ram may be kept in splendid shape. He can be used for two seasons on the ewes in one flock, and then when a change has to be made so as not to inbreed him on his own get, if he has been cared for properly, he will sell to another breeder for about his original cost, or very little less. Mangels and sugar beets should not be fed to rams or wethers, as stated elsewhere in this work.

THE EWE FLOCK.

When the flockmaster intends to raise sheep for mutton and wool production only, a grade flock should be established. By using a good pure-bred sire and retaining some of the best ewe lambs in the flock each year to take the place of the older ewes that are annually culled out and sold to the butcher, a fine grade flock may be developed in the course of four to five years. When a person desires to raise pure-bred sheep and sell them for breeding purposes the ewes selected for this work should be, like the ram, of the highest type, and best build and conformation for that particular breed. One may select pure-bred sheep of any kind to establish a flock, but if he fails to select the up-to-date type of the breed he chooses, he will soon learn when it comes to selling for breeding purposes that he cannot command the highest prices on account of lack of type. Likewise, if good type is in evidence, and the right conformation is lacking, the same thing happens. In raising pure-breds, start right, and you will always be right.

It has been stated that it is a mistake to use a ram lamb for breeding. However, it is a more serious mistake to breed the ewe lambs. First, one cannot raise fifty per cent of the lambs from ewe lambs, since nature has not fitted them to become mothers at this early age. Lambs born from ewe lambs are generally small and weak, and in spite of good care and feeding, the mother too often is not supplied with enough milk for the young lamb. Second, if the flockowner follows the practice of breeding ewe lambs, he will find in a few years that his flock is degenerating in size, constitution, and weight of fleece. These are all points worthy of consideration if success in sheep husbandry is expected.

CHAPTER II.

GENERAL MANAGEMENT OF THE FLOCK.

THE HANDLING OF SHEEP.

Many flockowners in this country treat their sheep simply as scavengers on their farms, but in England, however, they are handled in an entirely different manner. There the people treat their sheep as they should be treated, for they have had many years of experience in sheep husbandry and have learned to appreciate the value of sheep on the farm far more than do many people in America. Some men in this country handle their sheep in a manner that is cruel and really inhuman. The late Prof. John A. Craig, a friend of the writer and well known as one of the foremost authorities on sheep husbandry in America, while once watching sheep shearers at a large plant in the West, was witness to the cruelty of some of the brutal shearers toward the sheep. During a short time in their careless and reckless haste they slashed open the bellies of three sheep so badly that their intestines ran out on the shearing floor and the sheep had to be killed in order to relieve them of the terrible pain they were suffering. And yet we speak about humanity!

The writer himself could mention many instances of such cruel and barbarous handling of sheep that he himself has been witness to, but

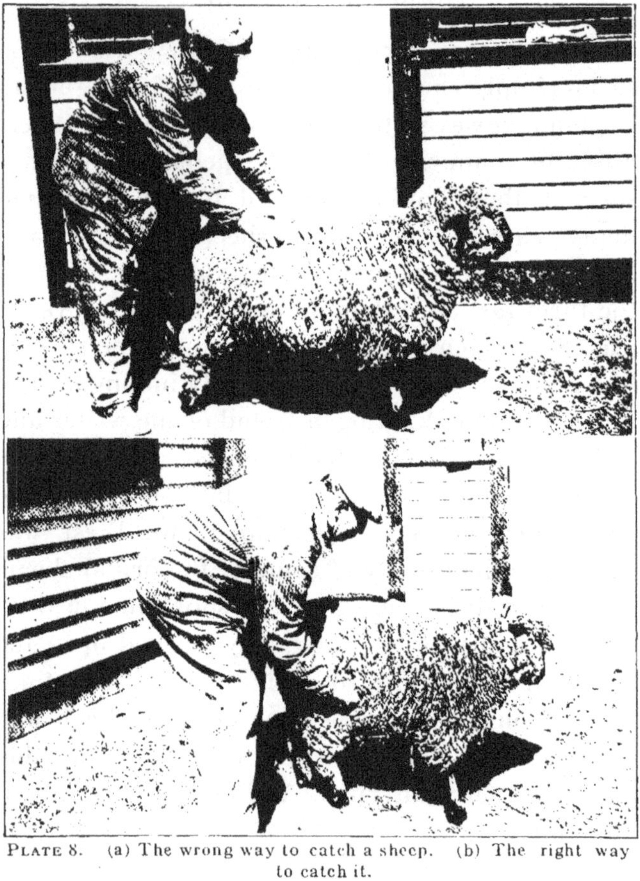

PLATE 8. (a) The wrong way to catch a sheep. (b) The right way to catch it.

these things have been done and cannot be altered. Nothing will be said here about the starvation of so many poor sheep on the Western ranges during the winter months. Let us at least learn to pick up those pieces of barb wire, broken from fences, that lie across our lanes, so that sheep will not daily get tangled, cut their legs, and pull out their wool. To get all the profit which is possible out of sheep many such matters, which may seem like trifles, must be attended to by the shepherd.

CATCHING THE SHEEP.

When the shepherd wishes to catch a sheep he should grasp it at the proper place, namely, at the flank. The accompanying illustrations show the wrong and the right way to catch a sheep. Many an ignorant flockowner catches and takes hold of the sheep by the wool, at any place he can get hold of best, in the manner shown in the first picture. Men who do this do not realize that the skin of the sheep is very lightly attached to its flesh, and that by holding the sheep by the wool in this careless manner the skin is torn loose from the flesh as far and a little farther than the hand's reach, thus injuring the innocent sheep. It has been our experience that it takes the sheep about two months to recover from the bruise thus caused. On the other hand, if the sheep is held by the flank, as is shown in the second illustration, no injury whatever is inflicted, and the largest and strongest ram will yield and stand still when caught in this manner.

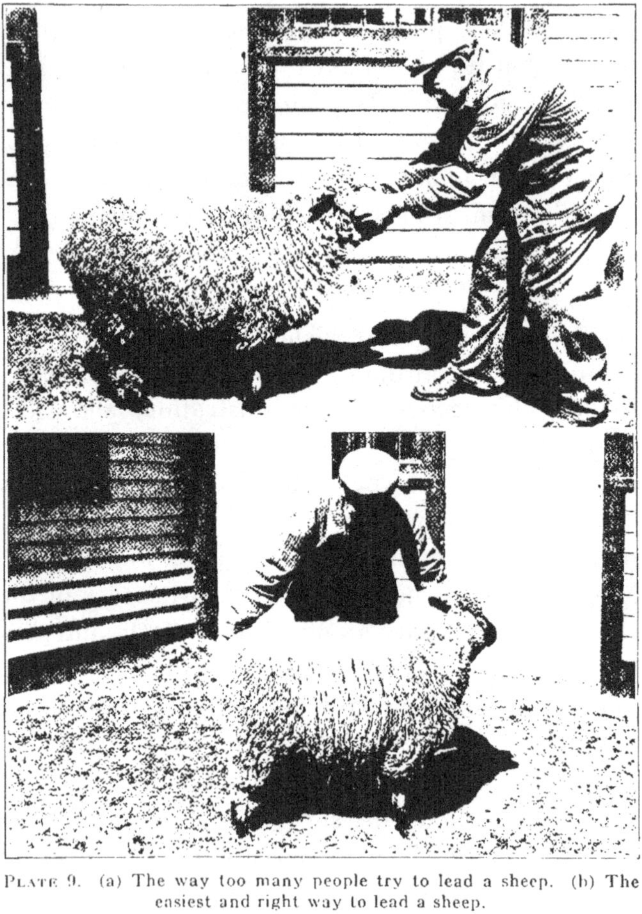

PLATE 9. (a) The way too many people try to lead a sheep. (b) The easiest and right way to lead a sheep.

LEADING THE SHEEP.

We often see farmers trying to lead a sheep by taking hold of it by its neck, of course also by the wool, and dragging it along. They make a hard task of it for themselves, and they certainly make it most unpleasant for the sheep. When properly handled all breeds of sheep lead fairly well, with the exception of the fine wools. These are more stubborn than the rest, but yet any breed may be led if the proper method is pursued. If a sheep is to be led, get on its left side, just the same as if you were going to lead a horse or cow. As is shown in the accompanying illustration, place your left arm around its neck, and your right hand on the end of its tail-head, tickling it just a little there, and you will find that it will, as a rule, come your way very quickly, or at times even faster than you care to have it come.

CARRYING AND LIFTING SMALL SHEEP OR LAMBS.

Occasions often present themselves when it becomes necessary to carry small sheep or lambs for a short distance, or to lift them from one pen into another. This work may be very easily performed by lifting the animal in the following manner: Standing nearly at the rear of the sheep, though slightly more to the right side, slip the right hand back of the sheep's right front leg and place it on

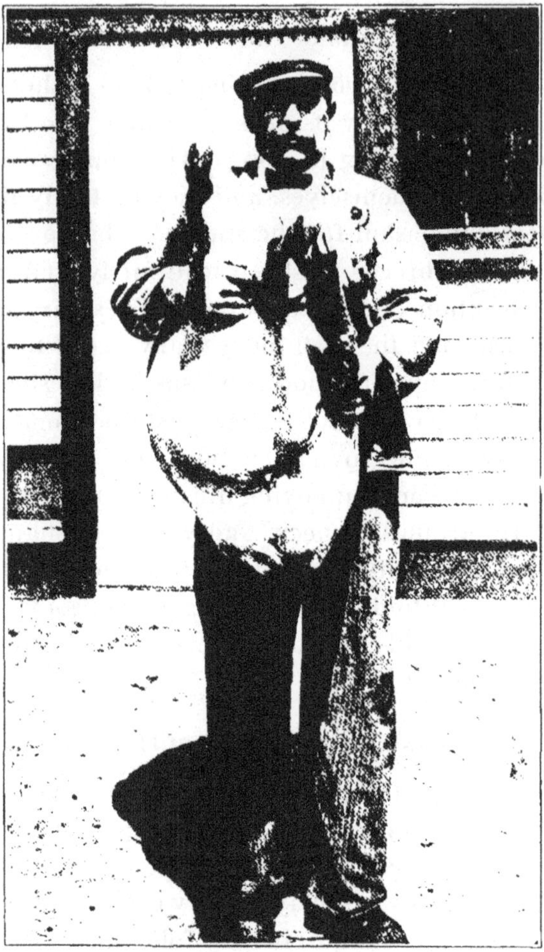

PLATE 10. An easy way to carry a lamb or small sheep without its struggling.

the brisket between the two front legs. Now lift the sheep slightly from the ground with the right hand to prevent its going forward. Then with the left hand take hold of the left hind leg just above the hock and lift the sheep up against your breast, as is shown in the accompanying illustration where a 108-pound lamb is being carried. By this method all struggling is avoided and no harm whatever done to the sheep.

SETTING A HEAVY SHEEP ON ITS RUMP.

It is a relatively easy task to set a light sheep or lamb on its rump by simply lifting it up and setting it down on its rump. However, with larger and heavier sheep, and especially with rams, it means a little more work and care. Perhaps the easiest way is to place the left arm around the sheep's neck, reaching back with the left hand and placing it firmly on the right forearm of the sheep. Now reach across under the sheep with the right hand, taking hold of the right hind leg just above the hock. Then the operator should shove against the sheep with his breast, and by pulling gently with the hand on the right hind leg, the sheep will be turned on its rump gently and easily, as is shown in the illustration which follows. When a sheep is to rise from this position some men will allow it to roll over on one of its sides and then let it struggle until it is finally able to get its legs under itself so it can rise. However, if the shepherd will push the sheep straight forward on its front feet when it is sitting on its rump, it will be able to rise easily and quickly.

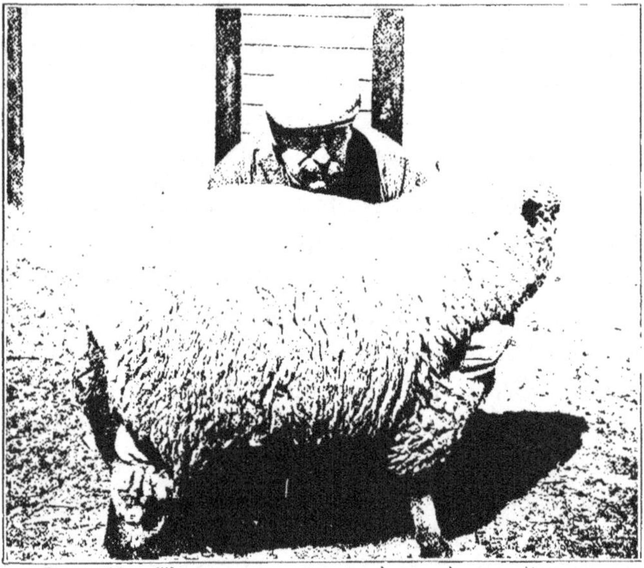

PLATE 11. The proper way to set a heavy sheep on its rump.

SORE TEETH.

When sheep show irregularity in eating or chewing their cud an examination of their teeth becomes necessary. The mouth of a sheep can be opened by means of two pieces of cloth, each about two feet long and two inches wide. One of these should be tied on the upper jaw, the other on the lower jaw between the front and back teeth. By pulling on these two strips one man will be able to hold the mouth open while another examines it, as is shown in the accompanying illustration.

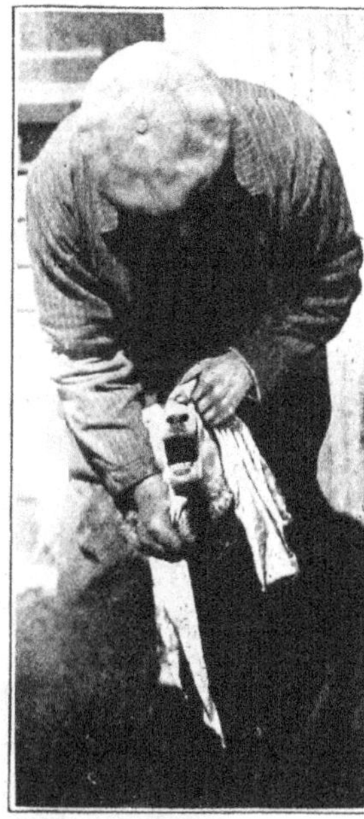

PLATE 12. How a sheep's mouth is held open while the teeth are being examined.

In case there should be a loose or badly decayed tooth that troubles the sheep in eating, this should be removed by means of a small pair of pinchers. If the outside edge of one of the back teeth has grown so long and sharp that it cuts into the flesh, a file should be taken and the sharp edge or point filed off. Many sheep have suffered from sore teeth without their owners knowing what ailed them.

THE AGE OF SHEEP.

The age of a sheep can be closely determined from its teeth. When a sheep has a full set of

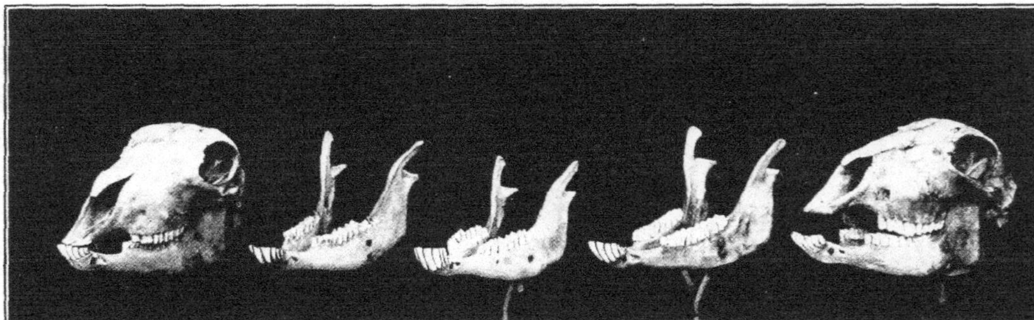

PLATE 13. The different ages of sheep, as shown by the front teeth. (a) Lamb's skull, all milk teeth; (b) jaw of yearling, one pair of permanent teeth; (c) jaw of two-year-old, two pairs of permanent teeth; (d) jaw of three-year-old, only one pair of milk teeth left; (e) skull of four-year-old, all permanent teeth, or "full mouth."

teeth we will find eight of them on its lower jaw in front, but none on the upper jaw. In the illustration are shown views of the entire skulls and of the lower jaws of sheep of different ages. The lamb's skull at the left shows its full set of first or "milk" teeth. These milk teeth are uniform in size and shape, and are rather narrow. After the lamb has reached the age of from twelve to fifteen months the central pair of milk teeth drop out, and a much larger pair of permanent teeth, or incisors, take their place. The second view shows the front teeth of a sheep of this age. At the age of two years another pair of milk teeth, one on each side of the first pair, will be replaced by another pair of permanent ones, as is shown in the third view. A year later the third pair of permanent teeth will appear, and only one pair of milk teeth will be left, as is shown in the fourth jaw. At length when the sheep is about four years old, the whole set of milk teeth will have been replaced by a full permanent set, as is shown in the last view.

We often find that the changes of teeth are somewhat irregular. For instance, the writer has seen rare cases where sheep did not change the first pair of teeth until they were eighteen and in one case nineteen months old, and then shortly after the first change had occurred the second took

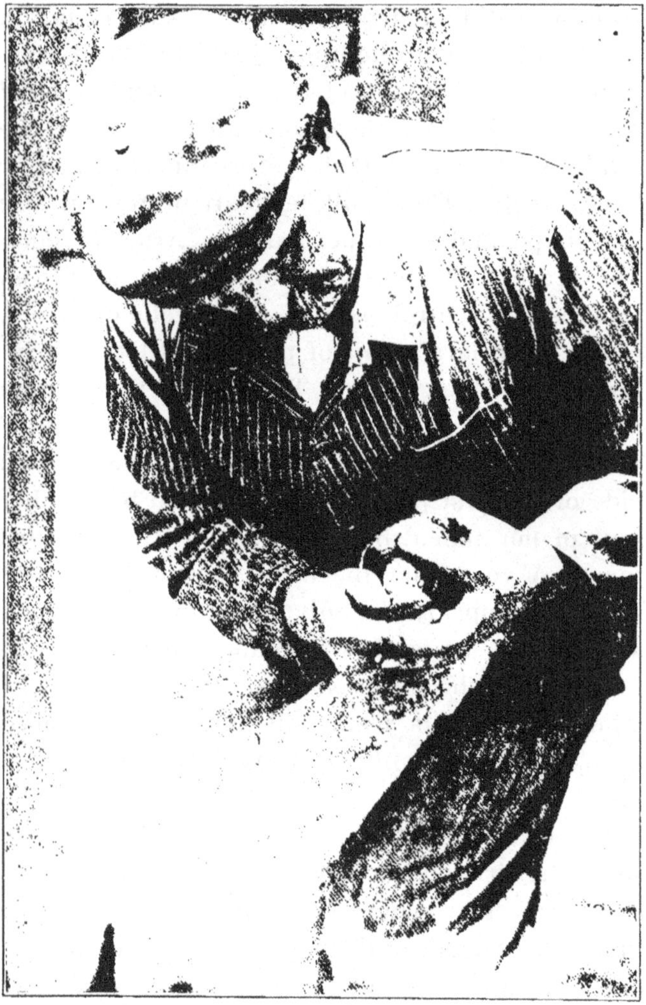

PLATE 14. The right way to part a sheep's lips to determine the age.

place long before the sheep was two years old. Heavy forcing in feeding will often hasten the early changing of the teeth.

At about four years of age, when the last pair of milk teeth has been replaced and the sheep has its full set of permanent teeth, the teeth will again be found more uniform. They will now be nearly as uniform as the full set of milk teeth the lamb had at first. However, the permanent teeth are all larger than the milk teeth and may be worn so that the corners are rounded off or the tops flattened, while the milk teeth are sharp and square. From the time the sheep is a yearling until it reaches the age of four years we do not find uniformity in the size and shape of the teeth, as there are always some of the permanent and some of the milk teeth present, and the latter are narrower and comparatively smaller than the permanent teeth.

After the age of four years no one can tell the exact age of a sheep by its teeth. However, well-experienced men can guess pretty closely by the looks of a sheep's face whether it is a five, seven, or eight-year-old. Many times the seven or eight-year-old has lost some of its teeth, or they may be loose in the mouth.

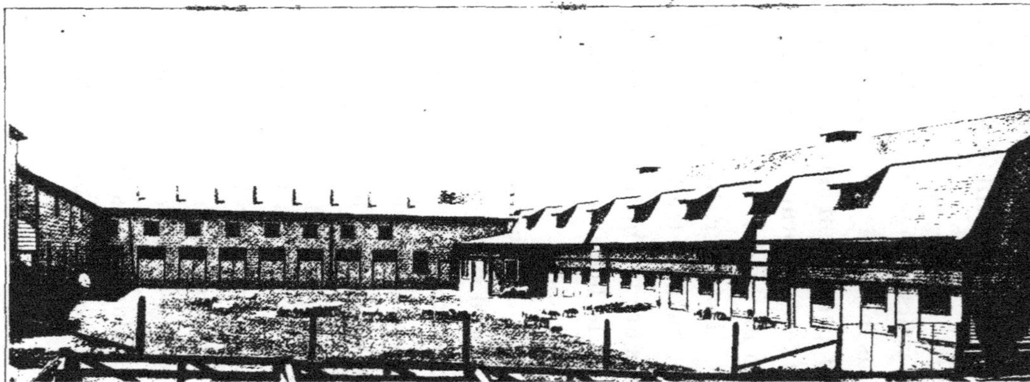

PLATE 15. Sheep barn at the University of Wisconsin. This barn was built especially for experimental purposes. Under a portion of the building is a root cellar, a part of the first floor is used for a general and private office of the man in charge, while the upper story is used for the storage of hay and bedding and contains a sleeping room for the shepherd. As a rule sheep do not require an expensive barn, especially if the ewes do not lamb until late spring. A common shed, with a hay or straw roof, will often answer the purpose. (Page 37).

CHAPTER III.

WINTER CARE AND FEEDING.

WINTER GRAIN FOR THE EWE FLOCK.

Sheep will thrive on the grains and roughage which are grown on the average farm. Breeding ewes that come into winter quarters in good condition do not need a great deal of grain. The flockowner should aim not to let them run down in condition, as is often done. Wherever breeding ewes are forced to go through a process of starvation in the winter time great loss and all sorts of trouble appear toward spring and lambing time. While breeding ewes should not be poor in condition, it is also a mistake to have them too fat. However, if the writer had to make a choice between the two conditions, he would prefer the latter.

A mixture consisting of one and one-half parts oats and one part bran has given very satisfactory results when fed to pregnant ewes. The oats strengthen the ewes, and the bran is laxative and serves to keep the digestive organs in good working order. All fat producing varieties of grain, such as corn, barley, rye, oilmeal, and cottonseed meal, cannot be recommended to be extensively fed to pregnant ewes, since they have a tendency to produce a surplus amount of fat inside of the body, and thus make it difficult for the lamb to develop properly. When ewes are fed extensively on these rich grains, in many cases their systems are heated up and they shed more or less of their wool long before shearing time.

AMOUNT OF GRAIN TO BE FED.

No man can lay down a definite rule as to the amount of grain to be fed to a sheep per day, since they vary in size and condition. It has been found that one-half pound per day of the grain mixture already mentioned is sufficient for a medium sized ewe, weighing from 150 to 170 pounds, during the winter months. When good alfalfa or clover hay is fed, in conjunction with some succulent feed, no grain is needed up to about one month before lambing time. At this time, however, it becomes necessary to feed some grain in order to insure a good milk flow for the young lambs.

SUCCULENT FEEDS.

All succulent feeds tend to keep the bowels of sheep in excellent condition, and have a general tonic and regulating effect. Chopped roots are as good a succulent feed as can be recommended. They may be chopped up by means of a root pulper, which can be purchased at small cost and is very useful. Among all the varieties of roots grown the writer in his experience has found rutabagas the most satisfactory for sheep feeding. While roots are very good for sheep feeding, although somewhat expensive to grow, there is another succulent feed, namely corn silage, that will take their place, for sheep relish good sweet corn silage. Care should be taken when feeding silage that no spoiled or moldy stuff is fed, which is very detrimental, nor sour silage, which contains a great deal of acid and causes colic, stretches, and scouring. All such silage is dangerous, especially to pregnant ewes, as it is apt to cause abortion. Such poor silage fed to ewes after lambing will also cause the suckling lamb to scour, often resulting in death. Good succulent feeds are, however, very essential for breeding ewes after lambing time, as they increase the milk production for the lambs. It is not a safe plan to feed too much succulent feed to pregnant ewes, as it would be responsible for what are termed large, soft, flabby lambs, which have no strength or vitality when born and ultimately die. It has been learned at this Station that two pounds of succulent feed (roots or silage) can be fed safely per day to a pregnant ewe with good results. After lambing time this amount can be increased. Care must be taken that no frozen roots or silage are fed, for some sheep feeders have experienced bitter losses of sheep after feeding frozen roots or silage. Frozen roots chill the stomach, while frozen or moldy silage may have a poisonous effect. Either will cause a serious derangement of the digestive organs.

ROUGHAGE FOR SHEEP IN WINTER.

Sheep like variety in their feed, perhaps more so than other farm animals. Alfalfa, red clover, and other leguminous hays are their favorites. Oats and peas sowed together and made into hay before they ripen make an excellent winter feed for sheep. Blue grass hay, oat hay, nice corn fodder, and bright, fine oat straw are also relished by sheep as a change. Timothy and marsh hay should at no time be offered as feed to sheep. Too much emphasis cannot be placed upon this statement, for timothy hay with its coarseness and woodiness has caused the loss of thousands of sheep annually in this country from constipation. Another objection to timothy hay feeding is the fact that the heads of the timothy force themselves into the wool, often down to the skin, making the skin itch very badly and causing the sheep to scratch and rub on sharp corners. The timothy in the wool also makes shearing difficult, and wool buyers object to such wool and cut down on the price paid for it.

WINTER QUARTERS FOR SHEEP.

Winter quarters for sheep should be of such a kind that the sheep are dry above and underfoot. Therefore, when a sheep barn or shed is built it should be properly located. If possible, a spot of elevated ground should be selected to provide good drainage on all sides. There should never be a time when water runs into the sheep barn during heavy rains or when snow is melting rapidly in winter. When sheep are forced, contrary to their nature, to lie down on a wet floor in a barn rheumatism and stiffness in legs and body will soon set in. Though sheep like dry quarters in winter they do not prefer too warm a place, as their coat of wool keeps them sufficiently warm. Another important factor leading to the welfare of the flock is to avoid all draughts. Coughing, running at the nose, and lung diseases are often due to draughts sweeping through the barn or shed. The barn should be dry, airy, and well-ventilated, but must be free from draughts. It should also be well lighted, since sheep prefer the light and thus do not thrive so well in a dark place. The barn must have wide doors, so that the sheep do not get jammed and injured by rushing through too narrow doorways. The results of narrow doorways are broken-down hips, the squeezing and crushing

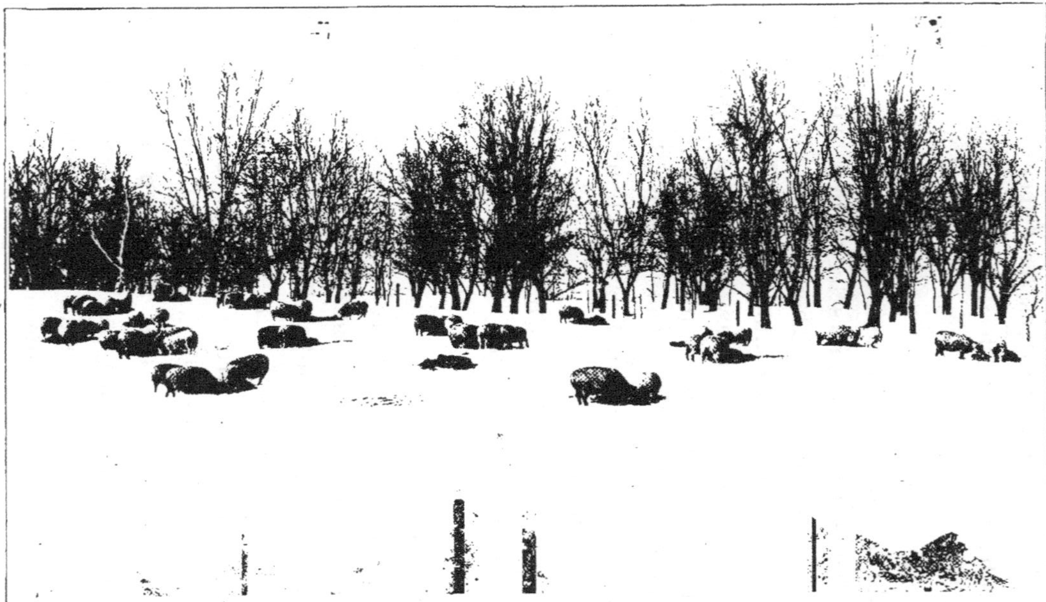

PLATE 16. There is no better way to excerise the pregnant ewes during the winter than to scatter their roughage in small piles in the field. When the snow is deep, a path can be made for them with a snow plow

of little lambs, and the abortion of ewes heavy with lamb.

Again, plenty of room should be provided for sheep. A close, cramped condition is very dangerous, especially for pregnant ewes. Some authorities say that from eight to twelve square feet are not too much room for each breeding ewe. Of course the amount of space allowed each ewe will depend somewhat on the size and breed.

LAMBING PENS.

Most sheep breeders provide a separate enclosure in the sheep barn which is divided up into several small pens called "lambing pens." In these are placed the mothers with their newly born lambs, each family by itself. These lambing pens are of great value when lambs are born in the cold winter months, February or March, and prevent much annoyance from ewes disowning their lambs.

EXERCISE FOR SHEEP IN WINTER.

Too much emphasis cannot be placed on the importance of exercise for pregnant ewes. The more they walk and move about the stronger and healthier the lamb crop will be. If pregnant ewes have lots of exercise they will deliver their lambs more easily, and to a great extent this will prevent the lambs from coming wrong end first. The best and most satisfactory way to get them to exercise freely is to haul their roughage out into the field and spread it in small bunches, so that they will have to run from one place to another to pick it up. John Miller, a very prominent and successful sheep breeder in Canada, makes it a point to have his breeding ewes walk two miles every day when the weather permits. They leave the home farm in the morning and walk to an adjoining farm one mile distant where the hay is fed, and then return again in the evening.

On all days when the weather is favorable, breeding ewes should be out of doors for exercise. On all wet, rainy, or stormy days sheep should never be turned out. The flockmaster must exercise judgment in this respect. To let the sheep get their fleeces soaking wet in the winter time is a grievous mistake. There is not enough warm sunshine in winter to dry them out again, and sheep carrying wet coats on their backs are liable to contract colds or pneumonia, which may result in death.

Some sheep owners allow their breeding ewes to exercise by picking on straw stacks. This method is not advisable, as a great deal of chaff, dirt, and other material gets into their wool. Others force their sheep to make their entire living all winter long from a straw stack. Such men as these cannot expect their ewes to furnish much milk for their lambs when born, nor shear a heavy, clean fleece of wool. Some winters when a deep snow is on the ground it is difficult to get the ewes out from the barn any distance at all. Where a snow plow is kept on the farm a path can then be made out into the field for sheep to follow. If such a plow is not available two ten or twelve inch planks may be fastened together, like a stone boat, the front end being pointed. A horse may then be hitched to them, and the driver by standing on the planks can make a path wide enough to let the sheep pass through. By all means exercise the ewes in some manner, in order to insure a good lamb crop, for the good shepherd spares no effort in promoting the health and comfort of his breeding flock. The careless one depends largely upon the season and so-called "good luck," but good luck is a result of good judgment and good care. The returns in both cases are proportionate to the effort and care given.

The best shepherds in this country claim that sheep should not be allowed to become wet from about November 1 to May 1. On the days in winter when the cold northwest winds are sweeping over the country, and when the wind almost cuts a man's face, sheep are much better off if kept in the barn. When exposed to these sharp, cold winds

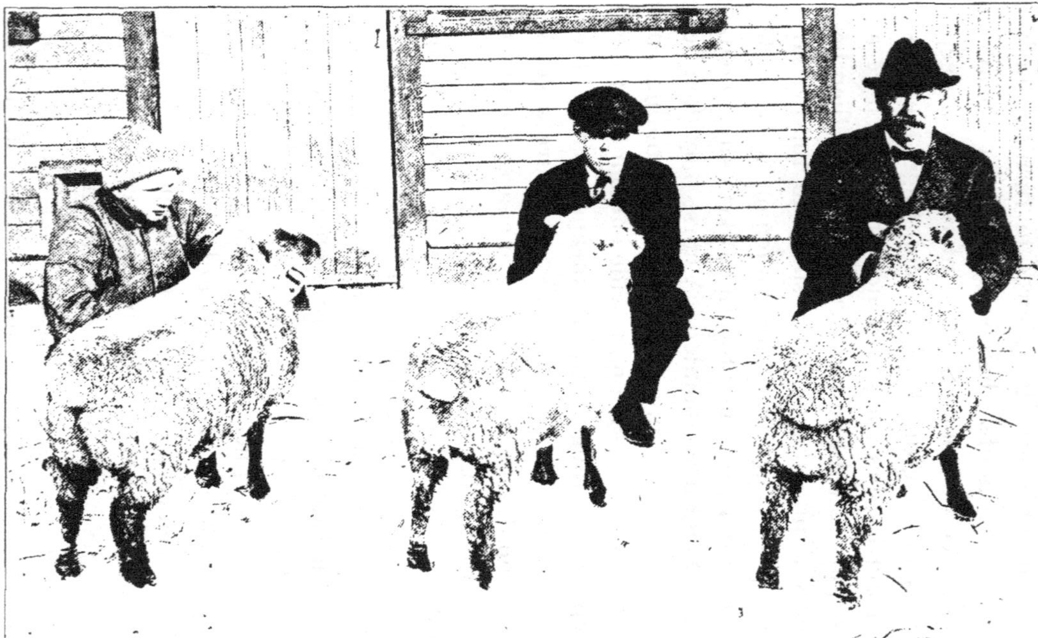

PLATE 17. Pure-bred Southdown wether lambs. First prize lamb at the right; third prize at the left; also winners of the first prize pen of three wether lambs at the International, 1917, shown by the University of Wisconsin.

their eyes are affected, a white film covers them, and they become blind. It is often from two to three weeks before their eyes get well, and many flockowners have been quite alarmed at this trouble. Sheep that are affected in this way should be isolated from the flock and kept in the barn, not in a draught, until their eyes get well. A few drops of raw linseed oil put on the sore eyes once a day will help them heal.

GESTATION PERIOD OF EWES.

Records have been kept at this Station which show that the length of time that ewes carry their lambs varies considerably. These records have been kept for all the breeding ewes in the Station flock, including many different breeds. The date of service of each ewe, as well as the date of lambing, has been recorded. These records, which extend over a period of about twenty-four years, show that the fine wool breeds seem to require a longer gestation period than other breeds. Next to the fine wools may be placed the Cheviots. The average gestation period of about 1500 ewes on record was from 146 to 147 days. The largest per cent of ewes have lambed at 146 days. In many instances Merinos have required a period of from 150 to 154 days, and Cheviots in many cases a period of from 146 to 151 days. Whenever a ewe carried her lamb or lambs from five to seven days overtime the result was usually weak or dead lambs. After careful study and observation the writer has been led to believe that outdoor life and giving ewes all the exercise possible hastens the date of lambing.

The winter of 1910–11 was an unusually mild one in Wisconsin, especially in the southern part of the state. Because of this fine weather the Station flock of breeding ewes could be turned out into a field about a quarter of a mile away from the barn. Here the hay was spread so they had to pick it up. From the time that the ewes were bred until all had lambed they were turned out in this field daily on all but eleven days, when they were kept in on account of snowy or rainy weather. Our records for that year show that out of 60 ewes which lambed only ten carried their lambs from one to three days overtime. Four out of the 60 dropped their lambs on the proper day as given for them in Breeders' Memorandums, or so-called Breeders' Calendars, 147 days, while the remainder, 46 ewes, dropped their lambs at from one to five days ahead of 147 days. All lambs, whether dropped on or before time, were unusually strong and healthy. The record for that year is quite different from that of former years, when on account of more snow and bad weather the

Station flock could not get as much exercise and enjoy as much outdoor life, showing that the difference in the vitality of the lambs and the shorter time they were carried must have been due to the abundance of outdoor life and exercise the ewes had.

LAMBING TIME, THE SHEPHERD'S HARVEST.

Lambing is perhaps the most critical time of the year for the shepherd. At this season he is expected not only to be on strict duty during the day time, but must also sacrifice a good share of his night's sleep. The experienced shepherd knows that his success and the percentage of lambs raised depend in a great measure upon how closely he watches with his flock at lambing time. In England, for the sake of encouraging the shepherds to take the best care of their flocks and new born lambs, the owners pay an extra percentage for all lambs raised, in addition to the regular month's wages.

EWES WITH TWINS AND TRIPLETS.

As a result of proper mating and the thrifty condition of both ram and ewe at the time of breeding in the fall, a great many twins and even triplets may be expected. When the lambs begin to come, with their arrival all sorts of troubles present themselves, not nearly so many, however, with

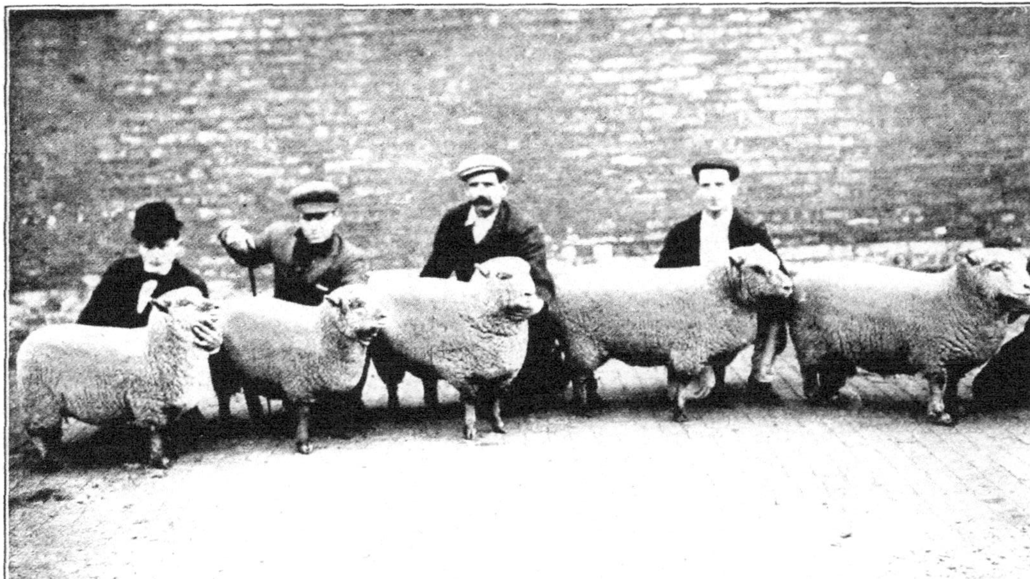

PLATE 18. First prize flock of Southdowns at the International 1910, shown by Charles Leet & Son, Mantua, Ohio.

the man who understands his business as with the man who is a beginner in the work. It is not wise to let ewes with twins or triplets remain with the whole flock. In fact, it is much better not to let any ewes remain after lambing with those that have not yet lambed, as the ones which have lambed need more feed. Ewes with twins or triplets, when left with other sheep, often disown one of their lambs. In the majority of instances the stronger lamb comes first, and soon after birth it looks for its first meal. Its mother, however, is in pains to deliver another lamb, and therefore she will not move away from the nest which she has selected for lambing, which is generally in one corner of the barn. Thus the mother does not follow her new-born lamb, but the other inquisitive sheep flock around to see the newcomer and often lead it away. The new-born lamb thus loses track of its mother, and the mother likewise loses the smell of her lamb and refuses to own it when she meets it again, since ewes recognize their lambs *only* by their smell and voice. Such ewes should, therefore, be put away separately either in the lambing pens or in a special place temporarily prepared for them by means of hurdles placed in corners in the barn. Here they can be kept for a couple of days until mother and lambs are thoroughly familiar with each other.

EWES WITH SINGLE LAMBS.

Ewes with single lambs often disown them on account of the lack of milk to support them, caused by the fact that they have not been properly fed before lambing. Young ewes that have their first lambs belong to this class in particular. Each ewe should be put by herself with her lamb and be fed grain and milk-producing succulent feeds to start the milk flow. The lamb which does not get enough milk from its dam should in the meantime be helped along by means of cow's milk until its mother is in shape to care for it.

LAMBS BORN WEAK.

Once in a while a lamb is born in a weak condition. The careful shepherd is on hand to assist it by lifting it up to its mother's udder, putting the teat into its mouth, and drawing some milk into the mouth with his fingers. This should be repeated until the lamb, after it has once had the taste of milk and has gained strength, is able to stand and drink by itself.

Some lambs, although they may be born strong, are unable to find the mother's teat. Ewes sometimes have their udders wrapped up in dense or long wool, which makes it difficult for the lamb to find the teat. This is especially the case with Shropshires and long wool breeds. In such instances the surplus wool should be removed at once with the sheep shears, and the lamb be assisted at its first meal. In rare cases it also becomes necessary to open up the teat by squeezing out the little wax in the end of it.

REVIVING THE ALMOST LIFELESS LAMB.

Often a lamb has a hard struggle at birth and arrives in this new world almost exhausted, lying without any signs of lung action. The shepherd has assisted the ewe in bringing the lamb forward, but it seems to be almost, yet not quite, dead. All that shows the lamb to be alive may be a single quiver. Now is the time when he must act quickly to revive the lamb. The first thing is to clean all phlegm out of its mouth, then he must hold the mouth open with his two hands and blow gently three to four times into it to start up lung action. Now he must lay it on its belly and beat it slightly with his two hands, one on each side on its heart girth right back of the shoulder, and if it does not commence to breathe, he should blow into its mouth again. If there is the slightest bit of life left in the lamb, he will revive the lamb by this method. Many such lambs that at first sight appeared to be dead, have been revived by the writer in this manner.

THE CHILLED LAMB.

It is a matter of fact that lambs have been born out of doors at a temperature down to zero and sometimes even below zero, and yet have come out all right. However, even the strongest lamb is liable to become chilled if it has to remain for a while in extreme cold. The best way to revive a chilled lamb is to give it a hot bath in a pail or tub of water as warm as the hand can well bear. After this bath take a piece of woolen cloth and wipe the lamb dry, which will tend to start up the circulation of its blood. Wrap the little one in a warm, dry piece of cloth and place it for a while near a warm stove. When it has come to, a little warm milk taken from its mother should be given it to encourage strength. A few drops of whiskey in a little warm water would be beneficial to the youngster. After it has gained sufficient strength it should be returned to its mother.

The lamb, however, needs to be watched for a few days as it becomes constipated from the effects of its chilled condition. If such be the case, from one-half to one teaspoonful of castor oil may be given the lamb, depending on its size. If one dose does not have the desired effect, one or two more should be given until the bowels move properly.

ADOPTED LAMBS.

If a ewe loses her lamb she may become a step-mother. A lamb may then be taken away from another ewe that has more than one lamb, and given to the ewe which has lost her lamb. This can easily be done by skinning the dead lamb and putting the skin on the lamb that is to be adopted. The odor of the skin of the dead lamb will make the ewe believe that it is her own. This skin must be removed in from 48 to 54 hours, or it may cause the lamb's own skin to decay.

Another way is to hold a ewe about every two to three hours and let the lamb suck, and she will own it in five or six days. The ewe that is to adopt the lamb should be put into a small enclosure or tied with a halter so that she cannot bunt the lamb, as otherwise she may kill it. The writer has often taken lambs that did not get any too much milk from their own mothers and has let them drink the surplus milk of ewes with an overflow.

NEWLY LAMBED EWES.

All newly lambed ewes should be examined for a few days, both in the morning and the evening, to see whether the lamb or lambs are taking all the milk out of the udder. It is peculiar that some lambs will only suck on one side of the udder, and the milk which is left on the other side will cake and spoil the udder. Often it takes a number of days for the lamb or even for two lambs to use up all the milk. All this surplus milk should either be taken by another lamb or should be milked out as long as necessary in order to keep the udder from caking.

ASSISTING THE EWE IN LAMBING.

In spite of the fact that the shepherd has given his flock the proper feed and an abundance of exercise, it sometimes happens that a ewe is absolutely unable to deliver her lamb or lambs. The ewe may have difficulty in delivering a lamb either because the lamb is unusually large, or because her passage way is too narrow, or because the lamb lies in the wrong position. Young ewes, lambing for the first time, have the most trouble in this respect.

When a lamb has come forward far enough so that its nose and front feet are at hand, but its head is unable to pass through, the ewe must be assisted. Sometimes the lamb can be brought forward by pulling on its front feet, but this alone will not in all cases be sufficient. It often becomes necessary for the shepherd to place one of his hands on the outside of the vagina right back of the lamb's head and press and squeeze the lamb's head through. Another good way recently discovered by the writer is to smear with the hand a lot of linseed oil on the inside of the vagina, especially where the lamb's forehead sticks. This will soften up the vagina and allow it to stretch, and will also make the passage way more slippery. The writer has had cases where he feared that the lamb could never be delivered without cutting the ewe open, but after using linseed oil in the manner described the lamb came forward at once with no further trouble.

If a ewe has passed the water bag and in about two to three hours does not show evidence of lambing, it becomes necessary to investigate the matter, as the lamb must be lying wrong, or be dead. Before investigating have your hands washed clean, and remove all long, sharp finger nails. Put a little carbolic acid or perhaps a little disinfectant, such as Zenoleum or Creso sheep dip, into some warm water, and scrub your hand and arm with it, so that they are thoroughly disinfected and clean before beginning the work.

Several different positions of the lamb may be the cause of non-parturition. The lamb may lie straight across the passage way, or with its front feet in the proper direction but its head turned back, or the hind end may come first and the hind legs under it; or perhaps one hind leg is forward and the other is backward. In the case of twins

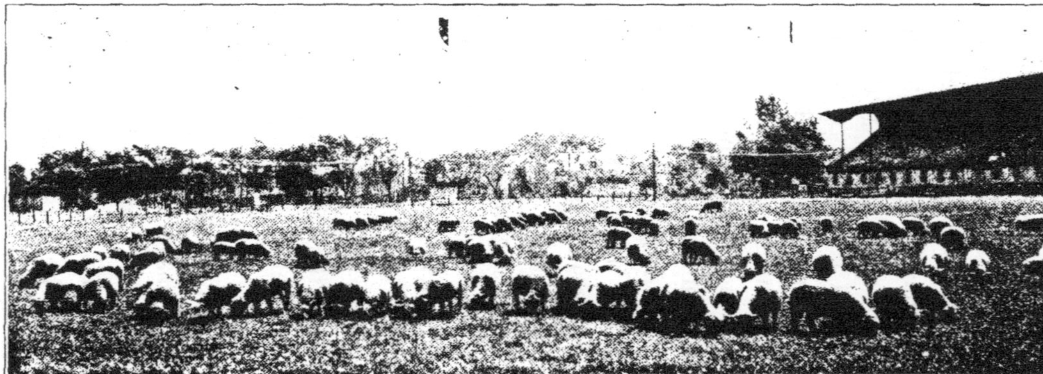

PLATE 19. Part of the University of Wisconsin flock "Hooverizing" on the University Athletic Field during the summer of 1917.

or triplets, the writer has seen cases where the legs and tails of the two or three lambs were entangled, forming a round ball, so to speak. In any of these cases the lambs will have to be taken from the ewe. A person with a small hand can do this work most successfully. After the operator has disinfected his hand thoroughly in order to pretect himself and the ewe against blood poisoning, and has softened his hand with sweet oil or lard, he will turn the lamb to its proper position, which should be head and front feet first in the passage way. He must exercise great care not to injure the ewe after he has inserted his hand in the womb, or inflammation will set in.

In some cases, the ewe with her natural pressure makes it impossible for the operator to insert his hand, and he may almost give up hope of saving the ewe and lambs. Yet at this critical moment the operator must not lose his head. Two men should be called in to assist him. Place the ewe with her head in a corner so that she cannot go forward. The two men will each now take hold of a hind leg around the thigh and elevate the rear of the ewe. This will hasten parturition. The pressure by the ewe will then cease and the lamb or lambs that have been pressed forward up to the narrow passage will naturally, on account of the elevation of the rear end of the ewe, drop back

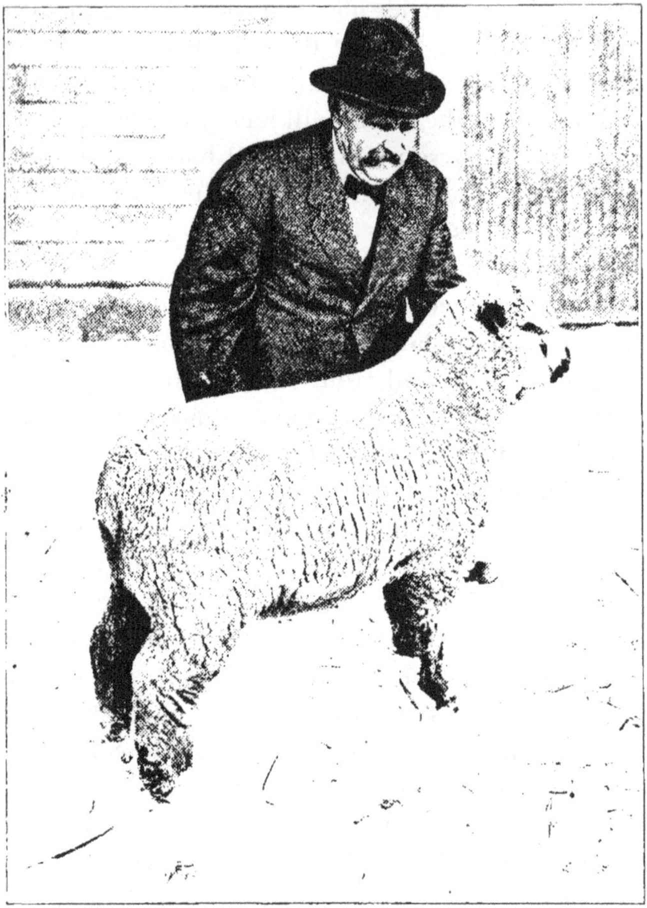

PLATE 20. Pure-bred Shropshire wether lamb. First prize winner at the International 1917, shown by the University of Wisconsin.

into the natural lamb bed. The elevation of the ewe prevents her natural pressure to a great extent, thus giving the operator a chance to untangle the lambs and turn them in the right direction and successfully bring them to daylight. After the lambs have been taken from the ewe the operator can take a lump of pure hog lard, the size of a hen's egg, and insert it in the womb of the ewe, where it will be very soothing and healing. The ewe may be given a tablespoonful of whiskey with perhaps a little gin to strengthen her. It may also be necessary to flush the ewe for two or three days once or twice daily by means of a rubber tube attached to a funnel, which is essential to prevent infection. For one application one-half teaspoonful of permanganate of potash should be dissolved in a quart of warm water. The above method of elevating the ewe should never be followed unless one is absolutely certain that parturition is possible in no other way.

FEEDING THE EWE AFTER LAMBING.

Some individual ewes in the flock are naturally heavier milkers than others, and this class is the most profitable to the owner. Where ewes have large udders the udders are very apt to become inflamed, and as a result the ewes will have milk fever if precautions are not taken with regard to their feeding. Draughts and lying on wet floors in barns are also responsible for this trouble in many cases. To avoid milk fever feed the ewe but little grain for three days after lambing. The danger of milk fever is over after this time, and the ewe may gradually receive her full allowance of grain again. Roughage and succulent feeds do not cause milk fever and may safely be fed both before and after lambing.

CAKED UDDERS.

A bad chill or cold, or a wet floor, as well as improper feeding, is enough to cause inflammation in the ewe's udder. The best remedy for caked udders is as follows: Upset the ewe and bathe the udder with warm water for about five minutes by means of a woolen cloth. When thoroughly bathed, gently rub it dry with a dry cloth, and rub in some melted pure hog lard, using it as warm as the ewe can stand. This should be done at least three times a day. Mercurial ointment, or so-called "blue ointment," can also be highly recommended. A hot woolen cloth held on the ewe's udder three times a day has also given good results. The milk that has caked in the udder must be milked out as thoroughly as possible each time the application of water and lard is made. Make sure that the ewe has nice dry bedding.

EWES WITH SORE TEATS.

Sore teats on ewes are generally brought about by the lambs. These youngsters often have very sharp teeth and in sucking not only bite the teat and make it sore, but also injure part of the udder. Ewes with udders in this condition refuse to let the lambs suck. When this state of things is first noticed milk out the milk from the udder at once in order to prevent clogging up and caking. Some vaseline should then be smeared on the sore spots at least three times a day until cured. Take a small file and file the front teeth of the lamb or lambs belonging to the ewe. File them down smoothly and make them somewhat flat on top, so that they cannot bite into the flesh and teats of their mother's udder.

TAGGING THE EWES AT LAMBING TIME.

All loose and filthy wool at the rear of the ewe should be clipped off, to prevent the lambs from biting it off and swallowing it. If ewes are not tagged and the lambs eat this filthy loose wool hanging about the dams it forms a sort of ball in the lamb's stomach, which stops the passage of the bowels and brings on death.

THE SHEPHERD'S ROOM.

On account of the dangers of lambing time it is most essential that the shepherd be near the flock at all times during this period. As a good shepherd must give up many hours of sleep in order to raise as large a percentage of lambs as possible, a small room should be provided for him in the sheep barn close to the lambing pens so that he may be comfortable during his weary watch. In this room should be a cot or bed upon which he can lie down when his duty does not require him to be with his flock. A stove should also be furnished so that the shepherd may keep warm in cold weather. By keeping a teakettle of water on the stove he will always have warm water on hand, which is often needed. Otherwise, if he should find a chilled lamb which needs a warm bath at once to revive it, he will be compelled to run to the house, build a fire, and warm water, causing serious delay.

Wealthy flockowners have even more furniture in the shepherd's room than is here mentioned. Good shepherds are always scarce, and if the flockowner is fortunate enough to have such a one he should make it as convenient and comfortable for him as possible during lambing time, his season of hardest work.

CHAPTER IV.

REARING THE LAMBS.

Young lambs usually begin to nibble and eat grain, or hay and other roughage with their mothers at the age of two weeks. At this time the lamb can be assisted by giving it some extra feed, in addition to its mother's milk and the little other feed it may get in the regular feeding trough with the older sheep. It is remarkable how these little fellows will grow if some extra grain and some nice clover or alfalfa hay is given them. A few roots saved up for the little lambs are beyond valuation for their growth and development.

The outcome and development of the flock depend largely upon the care the lambs get the first year. If the lambs are stunted then, they will always be stunted and will never make their proper growth. If once stunted as lambs, no matter how much or what kind of feed they may receive afterwards, their further development can not be greatly changed.

Another important factor which promotes the growth of lambs is to keep them in small groups in the barn with their mothers after they have been removed from the lambing pens. The writer has observed that these little fellows do much better when so treated than when a larger number is turned together when the lambs are still real young.

There is no other time in a sheep's life when it makes such rapid and economical gains as in its

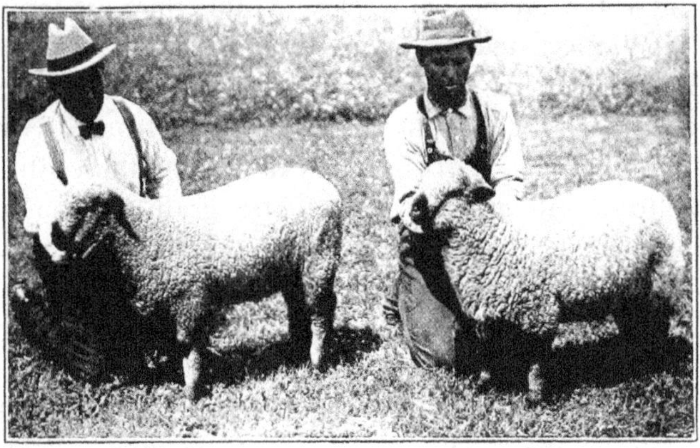

PLATE 21. Twin pure-bred Shropshire lambs at the University of Wisconsin. When three months old the ram on the left weighed 83 pounds, and the wether on the right 67 pounds.

first year, and especially so in the first six months after birth. At the Wisconsin Experiment Station the writer has raised many lambs that made an average gain of five pounds per head each week up to the age of three months. It is not at all uncommon for lambs to weigh fifty to sixty pounds when sixty days old. The accompanying illustration shows a pair of pure-bred Shropshire lambs, one a ram and the other a wether, raised at the Wisconsin Station. When three months old the ram lamb weighed 83 pounds and the wether 67.

The little extra grain, hay, and other feed consumed by young lambs is well repaid, and feeding young lambs grain has many advantages. Lambs born in March may be pushed ahead so that they can be sold in May or early June, when they will bring as much, or more, than they would bring in the fall. There is then a scarcity of nice, fat, plump spring lambs on the market, and as a rule, sell for exceedingly high prices.

On April 29 in the spring of 1910 at the Wisconsin Station we sold a grade Dorset lamb to a local butcher for fourteen cents per pound live weight. The lamb was forty-five days old and weighed forty-five pounds, bringing the sum of $6.30. A Hampshire was sold May 6, weighing forty pounds at forty-one days old, and bringing $5.60. Still another Hampshire was sold May 11, weighing fifty pounds at fifty-one days old, and brought $6.50 at thirteen cents per pound. If these same lambs had been sold at Chicago or New York a much higher price would have been received for them. At present, these prices would be doubled.

When lambs are fed extra grain and hay they do not suck their mothers down so in condition, as there is some substantial food in their stomachs and they do not have to depend entirely upon their mother's milk. It is a great pleasure to watch the little fellows eat and see them grow. The writer, engaged for many years entirely in sheep husbandry, has spent many five and ten minutes extra time outside of regular working hours, watching the little fellows assembled at the feed trough in the lamb creep enjoying their grain and nibbling some nice, bright hay and a few roots. If they should want more feed it is given them. It is just as much fun for the good shepherd to watch these lusty, growing, playful youngsters eat and play, as it is to watch a ball game.

For the person who is interested in sheep this is a very opportune time to learn sheep judging. The lambs are lined up close together, both large and small ones, and their build and general make-up can easily be studied at this time. There is one perhaps that is very wide at its hind quarters, but becomes narrower towards its shoulders, while right next to it there may be another one which illustrates exactly the reverse shape, being broad in front and narrow behind. One has a long neck, the other a short one; another perhaps has a hump back or looks as if its legs were crooked and too long, or has a little too much black wool on its head. Now let us look and see if we cannot find a few good ones among them, some that are about perfect. Perhaps at the middle of the trough we can see two or three, or maybe more, that look somewhat different from the rest. They are short-legged, blocky fellows, straight as a string on top, with sides from one end to the other just as straight and square as a timber coming out of a saw mill. They have short, thick necks, and carry nice, short, broad heads. The pleased shepherd realizes that they are unusually well-built lambs and will add some good material to his breeding flock and raise it to a higher standard. If perhaps he happens to be an exhibitor of sheep bright prospects loom up before him. He now feels assured that he has a good chance of winning some prizes with them at the county or state fairs, or perhaps even at the great International at Chicago. Remember, fellow sheepmen, that prize winners have to be built right, or rather, born right. Feed alone cannot and will not make them right.

THE LAMB CREEP.

The feeding of the lambs should be commenced just as soon as they will eat. This can best be done by means of a lamb creep, which can be set up at one side, corner, or end of the barn. The creep is very simple in construction and almost anyone can erect one. The material needed consists of two boards as long as desired and one inch thick and six inches wide, and also strips or slats, three feet long and one inch thick by four inches wide.

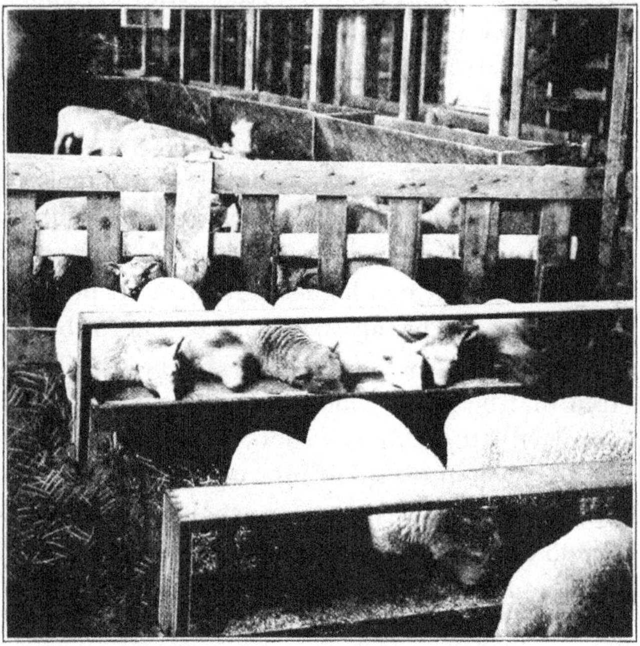

PLATE 22. Lamb creep and feed troughs in the sheep barn at the University of Wisconsin.

These strips are nailed on the two six-inch boards, thus forming a rack about three feet high. The slats should be put just far enough apart so as to let the lambs slip through and keep the old sheep out, as is shown in the accompanying illustration, which shows a lamb creep in the interior of the sheep barn at the University of Wisconsin. Within the space, thus set off specially for the lambs, is placed a feed trough, having a flat bottom. This

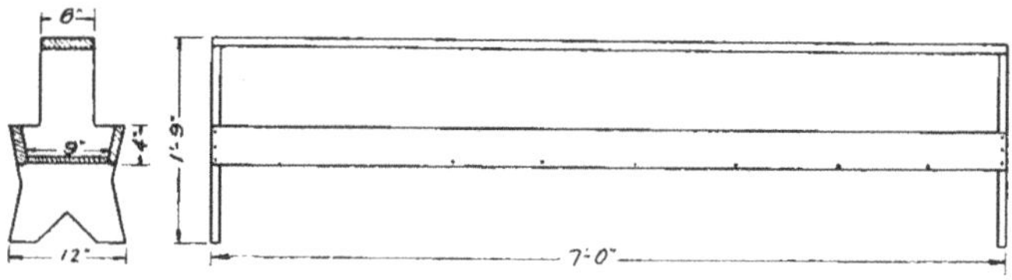

PLATE 23. Trough in which grain is fed to the young lambs.

trough is constructed in the manner shown in the cut. The trough is about four inches deep and nine inches wide and rests on legs nailed to each end. At each end of the trough a piece of six-inch board is nailed on, to stand up over the feed trough eight inches. On top of these two upright boards another six-inch board is nailed across the entire length of the trough to prevent the lambs from

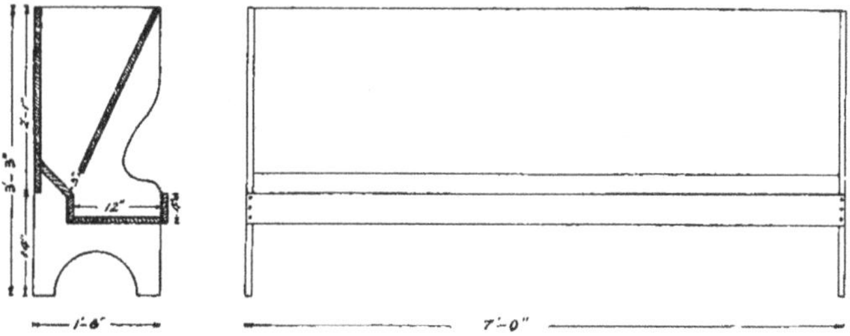

PLATE 24. Feed trough used at the University of Wisconsin, in which hay is fed to young lambs, and both hay and grain to older sheep.

stepping into it with their front feet. In this trough is put grain for the lambs. A simple and cheap hay rack, such as is shown in the cut, is used to feed the hay in. Young lambs are quite inquisitive, and when some grain and hay are placed in the creep, they will soon find the loop holes and begin eating.

GRAIN RATION FOR YOUNG LAMBS.

It has been found at this Station that a grain mixture consisting of two pounds of wheat bran, one pound of oats (whole oats will do, but crushed are better), one pound of finely ground cornmeal, and one-half pound of oilmeal has proved an excellent grain ration for young lambs. Later in spring when the weather gets warmer the amount of cornmeal may be reduced and the amount of oats increased. Fine second crop clover or alfalfa hay will furnish the best roughage for young lambs. If some roots, such as turnips or rutabagas, are available, the youngsters will soon relish them

When the sheep and lambs go out to pasture the lamb creep can be moved out with them and set up in a corner where the lambs will soon detect it again. Some sheep breeders may say that lambs do not need any extra grain when they are out on good pasture and are suckling their mothers. Experiments conducted along this line at this Station have shown, however, that it pays well to feed a little grain to lambs all summer long. Even if such lambs are held over for fattening in the winter it has been learned that the lambs fed grain during the summer make more and cheaper gains than lambs of the same breeding and kind that do not receive any grain while on pasture. If the lambs are fed well during their first year one can figure on a well-developed flock. There is no danger of getting them too fat, either for breeding purposes or for the butcher, if an excessive use of fattening grains is avoided. When well fed they grow so much that they do not lay on any surplus fat.

THE USE OF COW'S MILK FOR LAMBS.

Many people have made a failure of trying to raise lambs on cow's milk. Lambs may be successfully reared on such milk, however, if the proper precautions are taken in feeding. Young lambs are easily taught to drink cow's milk from a bottle with a rubber nipple attached to it, and after they have once tasted the milk they will quickly and freely run to the person carrying the bottle. Plate 25 shows how easily lambs may be taught to drink from the bottle. They may also be taught to drink out of a dipper. The reason why so many people have been unsuccessful in raising lambs by hand is in most cases that they did not understand the difference between cow's milk and sheep's milk as regards richness and fat percentage. People have a general idea that pure cow's milk is too rich for lambs, but the writer is of a contrary opinion. He knows from analyses

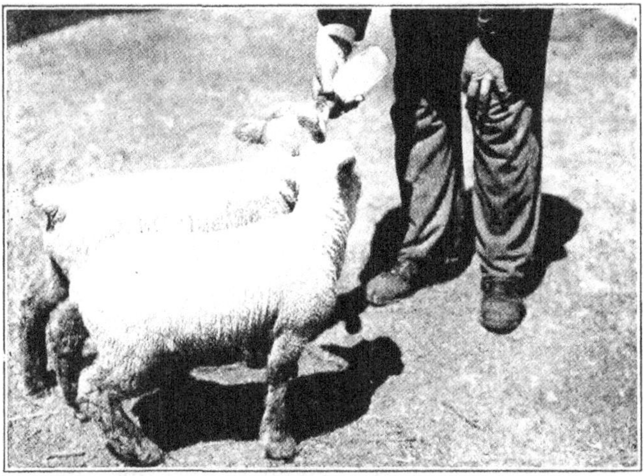

PLATE 25. One lamb is happy, the other wishes his turn would come. Pure-bred Southdown lambs raised on the bottle at the University of Wisconsin.

of sheep's milk that cow's milk is much lower in fat percentage than sheep's milk. Some years ago at this Station a grade Dorset ewe showed in a week's test 14.4 per cent of fat. Of course, her milk was richer than the average. It is astonishing to hear fairly well educated men say that one cannot feed cow's whole milk to lambs because it is too rich and will kill them. Such expressions of opinion seem laughable to the writer.

RAISING LAMBS BY HAND.

Raising lambs by hand is not generally a very profitable undertaking. Unless the lamb to be so raised is an exceptionally good one or a pure-bred, it hardly pays to spend the time required, especially considering the present high price of milk. The writer has, however, raised quite a number of lambs by hand, some of which made good and were prize winners at the International Show at Chicago. The lamb raised by hand has one advantage over its cousin suckling its dam. When the milk flow of the mother begins to cease the hand-reared lamb may still get a full measure of milk, and the amount fed can be increased as the lamb grows in size, providing plenty of milk is available.

There is more than one reason why some people have been unable to raise lambs by hand. One important reason is that they have not studied the instincts of the lamb and its mother. When the lamb suckles its mother it takes a little milk every little while, and this milk is warm and comes from a clean udder. When beginning to feed the young lamb on cow's milk the following points should be observed: First, the milk should be taken from a cow whose milk tests high in fat. Second, for the first three or four weeks the milk from this one selected cow only should be fed to the lamb. Third, for the first few days and nights the lamb should be fed every two to three hours, and a small amount (say two or three tablespoonfuls, with a gradual increase) given it each time, so as not to overload its stomach. Fourth, the milk should be warmed up to 92 degrees Fahrenheit, which is about the warmth of sheep's milk. Care must be taken not to let the milk boil as this causes constipation. Fifth, the bottle and nipple should be thoroughly washed each time after use so as to prevent the collection of sour matter in them, which in time may poison the lamb. When the lamb is first born it is delicate and has a rather weak stomach, and therefore great care must be exercised in rearing it by hand. Later on when it has become a month or so old the task is not such a difficult one.

MARKING THE LAMBS.

In all pure-bred flocks at least, all lambs should be marked, in order to keep the breeding records straight and to avoid mistakes when the time comes to have the lambs registered. It is a common statement among some sheep breeders that lambs should not be marked when very young, because the ear label, they believe, will make the lamb's ear hang downward instead of remaining erect. This idea is false. At this Station all lambs are marked either the first or second day after birth, and they surely carry their ears just as high and erect as if they had no label in them. Where

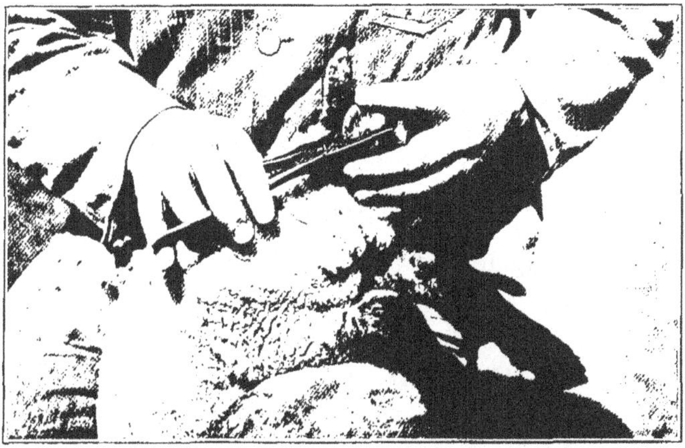

PLATE 26. Marking the lamb with the Dana ear label.

marking is done when the lambs are very young it saves the owner much time and prevents mistakes. It means a great deal of work later on to find the ewes and lambs that belong together if marking the lambs is postponed, and moreover mistakes may have already been made in registering such lambs. It is much better to mark them when young because of the time saved in doing so, and above all because of the assurance of keeping the record of breeding straight.

When inserting the label into the lamb's ear be careful to cut the hole between the veins so as to prevent bleeding. The Dana Ear Label has given very good satisfaction for marking lambs at this Station. The preceding illustration shows the manner in which the lamb is held when the marking is done. Another way to mark lambs is to tatoo their ears, but the writer does not consider this method nearly as good as using the ear label.

CASTRATING LAMBS.

No intelligent sheep breeder will allow his buck lambs to run without having them castrated. Only pure-bred buck lambs intended for breeding purposes are exempt from castration. The writer wishes he could use words strong enough to make those who have not operated on their lambs in the past appreciate the good results obtained from castrating them, and the evil results sure to follow when this is neglected. As a rule, at about the age of three to four months buck lambs begin to know that they are males, get restless, lose flesh, and as fall approaches become worse, jumping and riding each other, and hence getting in a thin condition, while castrated lambs get fat. When these buck lambs come to market in thin condition and with their testicles in them, which gives a strong taste to their meat, they will sell for $1.50 to $2.00 less per hundred pounds than lambs of the same age which have been castrated. Now flock-masters, is this difference in price not sufficient to set you to thinking and to make you decide to use the knife on your buck lambs in the future? At least the writer hopes that such will be the case.

METHOD OF CASTRATION.

Castration is not dangerous, if a little care is taken. Lambs can be castrated most easily and without much pain if the operation is performed when they are from one to two weeks old. Choose a nice, bright day, not a rainy, cold, or damp day. Select all lambs from the flock that are to be castrated, and fence them off in one end of the barn, providing it is done before going out to pasture. See that the barn is nicely bedded with clean straw. Mix a little disinfectant, such as carbolic acid or Zenoleum, in some clean, warm water, and disinfect your hands and knife in it. Then begin the work. First feel and make sure that both testicles have come down. Any lamb whose testicles have not both come down should be left alone until they have both come down. Cut off one-third of the lower end of the bag, pressing down firmly

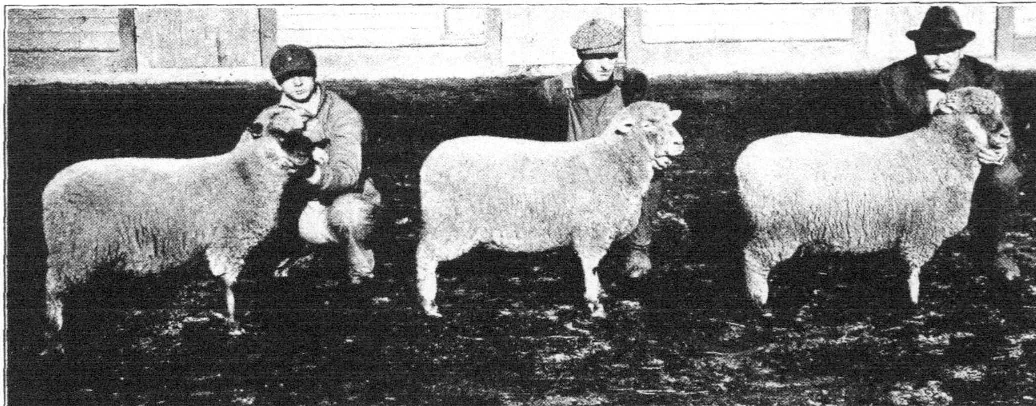

Plate 27. Pen of three grade ewe lambs. The result of using a pure-bred Southdown ram on western range ewes. The pen won 2nd prize in the mutton and wool demonstration exhibit at the International, 1917. Shown by the University of Wisconsin.

with left hand, which will leave the testicles partly exposed. Draw them out either with your fingers or a pair of pinchers. All fat and loose skin should be left in and worked back with one hand. The entire cord should be pulled out, *not cut off*. Pour a little disinfectant in the two holes from which the testicles have been removed, and then lift the lamb over the partition to its mother. The reason for fencing off the lambs is this: When lambs have been castrated they are unable to run, and generally lie down. If mothers and lambs are left together the lambs may get hurt by having their mothers run over them when the shepherd is catching other lambs. The operator can perform the neatest and cleanest job, if accustomed to do it, by pulling the testicles by means of his teeth. In nearly all foreign countries no lambs are castrated in any other way. If a lamb has grown quite old and the cord is too strong to be pulled it may be scraped off back of the testicle; this will prevent bleeding. Whenever possible, castrating the lambs should be done in the morning, and every disturbance of the flock should be avoided during that day.

DOCKING LAMBS.

All lambs should be docked, ewe lambs when they are from eight to fourteen days old, and ram lambs from five to seven days after castration.

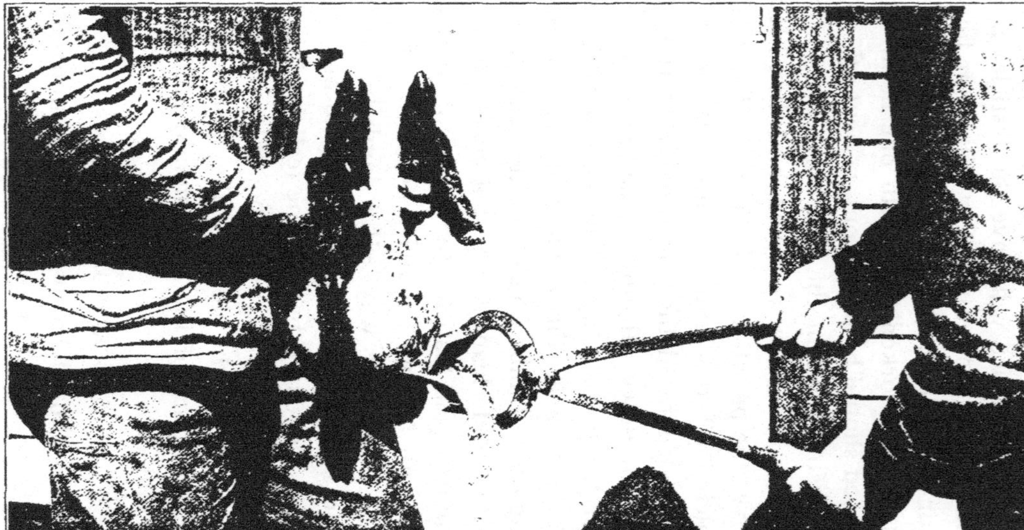

PLATE 28. How a lamb is docked with the hot pinchers.

When this is neglected flockmasters will suffer the loss of from twenty-five to fifty cents per hundred pounds on lambs when sold on the market, in proportion to the amount of dirt collected on the tails. We will not speak at all about the attractiveness of a bunch of lambs that are uniformly docked. Docking sheep prevents the accumulation of a great deal of filth at their rears, and consequently to a great extent keeps them from becoming infested with maggots, especially the females. The fact that many ewes do not get with lamb at all is due to their not being docked. Many flockowners are afraid to dock their lambs because they believe they will bleed to death. No danger need be feared, however, if the operator is at all careful.

There is more than one way to dock lambs. Their tails may be cut off with a sharp jack-knife. It used to be the custom to chop them off on a block by means of a chisel and mallet. When either of these methods is used the lambs lose blood, especially the fleshier ones, and in very many instances die from excessive bleeding.

If the lamb's tail is to be cut off the preferable way is to use a sharp knife rather than the chisel and mallet. One man must hold the lamb. The operator by feeling on the side of the tail can detect where the joints are. He should push the skin on the tail back toward the body of the lamb, so as to leave some surplus skin to grow over the stub, and then cut the tail at a joint about one and one-half inches from the body. This cut should be made so quickly with the sharp knife that the lamb scarcely knows that its tail is off. If any particular lamb should bleed too much a piece of cord or binding twine may be tied very tightly on its tail close to the body. This will put an end to the flow of blood, and the cord may be removed from the lamb in about eight to ten hours. Docking with the knife should be done in the morning, so that the lambs can be watched to see how they are getting along. The writer knows of some men who performed this work in the evening and the next morning found several of their lambs dead, due to great loss of blood. In cool weather nothing need be put on the wound, but in warm weather and in fly time some pine tar should be applied in order to keep the flies and maggots off.

Docking with pinchers is highly recommended. The plate on page 78 shows the method of docking a lamb with pinchers, and plate 29 shows a lamb which has just been docked. Ever since Joseph E. Wing invented these pinchers the writer has altogether abandoned the use of the knife for this purpose. By using the hot pinchers no danger need be feared from loss of blood. Older sheep than lambs can be very successfully docked with pinchers. While it is perhaps a little painful for the lamb at the time, if done rightly not a drop of blood is lost, and after a few hours the lamb jumps and runs about as if nothing had happened to it.

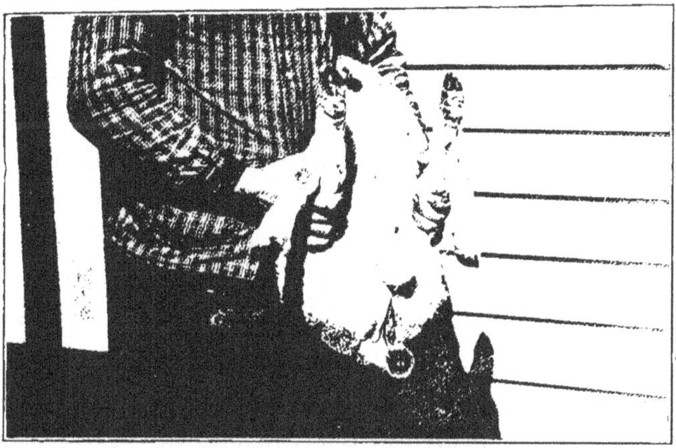

PLATE 29. The proper way to hold a lamb while it is being docked or castrated.

The pinchers can be heated nearly red hot in a common stove or in a blast torch, such as the tinsmith uses. Nine to ten lambs can be docked before heating the pinchers a second time. This method of docking is a great relief to the shepherd, since he does not need to worry for fear any of his lambs will lose too much blood and die. It also does away with all the squirting of blood over the barn and over the ewe's face and wool. There will also be no lost blood to be restored by feed, since it requires just so much blood to maintain a lamb. While the healing process of the tail is somewhat slower than if cut with a knife, nevertheless, taking all into consideration, this method proves more satisfactory in the end. In warm weather, just as in the case of cutting with the knife, put pine tar on the wound, in order to avoid maggots.

On the western ranges where large numbers of lambs are raised annually a general so-called "round-up" is made, at which castrating and docking is done at the same time. The ranchman saves time and labor in doing this work all at once, but this is no reason why the smaller flockowner should follow his example. When both operations are performed at once, it naturally gives the lamb a great shock and setback. The large flockowner of the West may perhaps save enough time by performing both operations at once to pay for the loss of lambs, especially since range lambs are not worth so much per head as the better grade of lambs owned on the smaller farms. The smaller flockowner, however, cannot afford to follow his example.

WEANING THE LAMBS.

The idea prevalent among flockmasters that lambs should wean themselves is in many ways not a good one. When a lamb has had its mother's milk from four and one-half to five months it is best to wean it. The breeding ewe is continuously laboring for her young from the time of conception, and if the lamb is not weaned from her before breeding time comes again she does not have a chance to rest at all. This rest, however, is very necessary for preserving her vitality and health. It has also been found that it is much better for the lamb to be weaned at the age of about five months. The lambs can then be turned on a fresh pasture by themselves where they do not draw any more parasites from the excrements of their dams.

The best way to proceed is to take the lambs away from the ewes, turn them on some fresh pasture, and not allow them to get back to their mothers again. Some flockmen allow the lambs to go back to their mothers after two or three days in order to remove the milk that has accumulated in the udder during the lamb's absence from its mother. This practice, however, is a poor one. Milk collected in the udder by a worrying ewe after her lamb has been taken from her is abnormal and has often done damage to the lamb.

Ewes and lambs find their first parting very bitter and they bleat for two days and nights until they finally forget each other. When the lambs are turned back again to milk out the ewes the old relationship is renewed, and it becomes hard for them to part a second time, to say nothing of the work of separating them.

CARE OF THE LAMBS AFTER WEANING.

When the lambs have been weaned they should have the run of some good, fresh pasture. The lambs will greatly enjoy grazing on land where one crop of hay has been cut and the new grass is coming up again, or on a piece of rape that has been sown in early spring. By turning them on new pasture the danger of stomach worms and other parasites is avoided to a large measure. Good, clean pasture is also necessary for them in order to avoid a check in their growth, as a result of the loss of their mother's milk.

CARE OF THE EWE AFTER WEANING.

After the lambs have been taken from the ewe great care must be taken to prevent the udder of the ewe from caking. Many mistakes are made in this regard. The best producing ewes in the flock are the ones that generally have their udders caked, for the reason that they continue to give

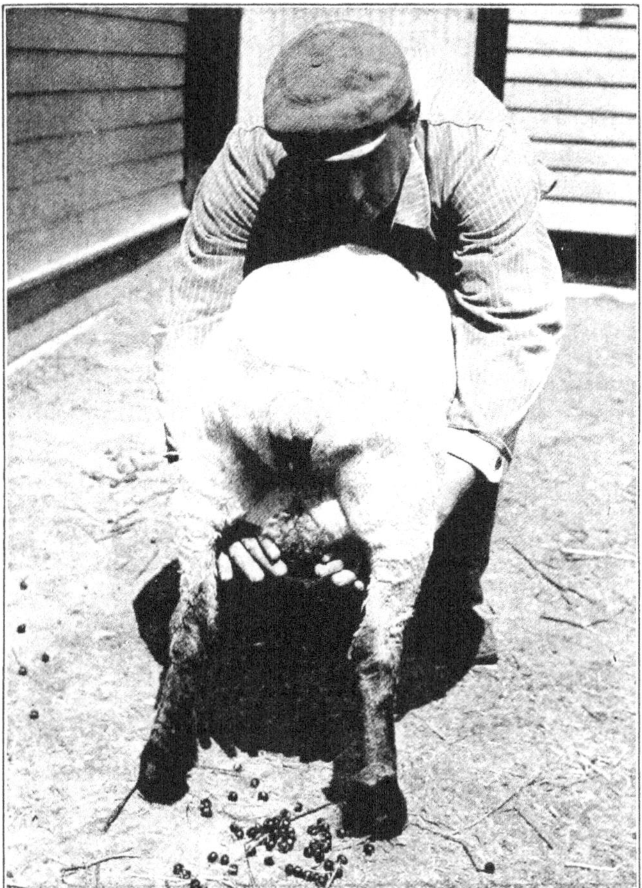

PLATE 30. Milking a ewe with two hands to hasten the work.

milk and this milk is not removed. While some ewes, as elsewhere stated, do not furnish their lambs very much milk at weaning time, others still have an abundance. Some ewes may be dried up in a few days, while others require a couple of weeks time to dry them up. In either case they should be given just as much attention as is given to cows when they are being dried off. The reduction in milk may be hastened along by putting the ewes on scant pasture for a few days.

The method of drying up ewes practiced by the writer is as follows: On a nice, cool morning when there is a prospect of having cool weather for a few days the lambs are all separated from the ewes. The ewes are then put on scanty pasture. The next day all the ewes are collected together in a fence corner in the field. One is caught and milked out, two hands being used to hasten the work, as is shown in the preceding illustration. Milking the ewe with two hands is accomplished by bringing her rear up against a fence, so she cannot go backward, and placing the two knees against her shoulders to prevent her from going forward. When partly milked out, just enough to keep the udder soft, she is turned loose and the next one is treated in the same way, and so on until all have been gone over. After two days' time they are again milked out in the same manner. Some ewes do not need any more attention after the second milking. Such ewes are marked on their backs with blue chalk to indicate that they are dry. Three more days should elapse before the next milking is done, and all those dry are check-marked. Another five days pass by and still a few more ewes have to be milked out. This is generally the last time they are milked out, with the exception perhaps of one or two who are extremely heavy milkers. In this way not a single udder will be spoiled.

GOITRE ON LAMBS.

This trouble which has resulted in the death of many lambs may be attributed to several causes. Perhaps, the pregnant ewe was fed too heavily on concentrated feeds, such as corn, cottonseed meal, barley, rye or even oilmeal. Succulent feeds, like silage, roots, or potatoes, if fed too heavily may cause a goitre. Keeping the ewes in closely cramped quarters, where it is warm and the ventilation poor, or not giving them enough exercise out-of-doors may also result in this condition.

For the lamb born with a large goitre nothing can be done. A goitre is occasionally formed on a grown sheep. Painting with tincture of iodine two or three times daily will often remove the goitre.

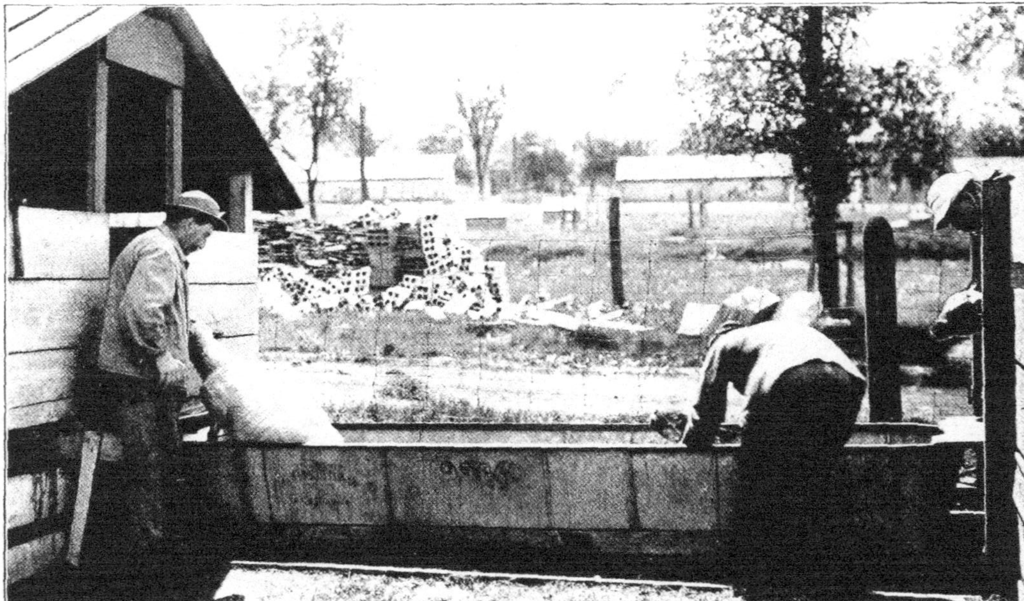

PLATE 31. Dipping sheep at the University of Wisconsin.

CHAPTER V.

SHEARING AND DIPPING THE FLOCK.

When warm weather comes on, flockowners should begin to think about shearing their sheep. In the Eastern, Middle, and Southern States, shearing commences about April 1 in most instances. Sheep in the Western States are, however, sheared somewhat later. Of course the time of shearing will depend largely upon the weather, the season, and the locality. Some sheepowners wait much later than the date mentioned for they know that when sheep are sheared real late in the season and after they have been on grass for a long time they have more yolk in their wool and hence shear a heavier fleece than when they are sheared early. The writer has known of cases where sheep were compelled to carry their heavy coats as late as the middle of June, through the hottest kind of weather, all because an increase of yolk and a heavier fleece were desired. It is true that the wool will contain more yolk when the sheep have been on grass for a long time previous to shearing, but there are disadvantages which more than counterbalance this fact. Often while flockowners are waiting for an increase of yolk in the wool the sheep will lose part of the wool on their bellies, necks and rears. Just as apples will drop off the tree when they are ripe, wool on sheep will fall off when ripe.

Moreover, when hot weather comes on while the sheep are still unshorn they will suffer greatly from the heat, and for this reason will lose flesh rapidly. When sheep are put on grass, owing to the resultant looseness of their bowels, their fleeces may get soiled, which lowers the quality of the fleece and also makes shearing disagreeable.

The cruelty of allowing the unshorn sheep to suffer from the heat should also be considered. It seems pitiful to see sheep lying by the side of a fence with their mouths wide open and tongues hanging out, panting and suffering from heat in the hot weather, simply because the owner is waiting for an increase of yolk and a heavier fleece. If flockmasters would only consider for a moment that the loss of flesh and body weight and the danger of the shedding of wool is far greater than any possible gain in yolk, then such foolish ideas would not so generally prevail. It is therefore clear that when the weather begins to get warm sheep ought to be freed from their heavy winter clothes, and an intelligent sheep breeder never thinks of waiting for more yolk. If sheep are fed as they ought to be during the winter, a good amount of yolk will surely be found in their wool when they are sheared, without waiting for grass to put yolk into it. Washing before shearing is no longer practiced since the woolen mills can clean the wool much better and more cheaply than the sheepman.

Shearing is now done mostly with machines, which are great improvements over hand shears. The shearing machine has the following advantages over the hand shears: First, the work is done more rapidly than with a hand shears; second, it is a neater and smoother job; third, sheep are not cut into nearly as much as with a hand shears; fourth, it is easier to learn shearing with the machine; fifth, using a shearing machine is not so hard on the shearer's wrist as using a hand shears; and sixth, a larger amount of wool is obtained because the sheep can be clipped closer. When a man is once familiar with the use of the machine he can shear many more sheep a day, and he can hardly be induced to go back to the use of the hand shears. A careless shearer should not be employed to shear either with hand shears or with a machine, for a rough, careless man can hurt the sheep badly by either method. Such a shearer, however, will cut the sheep worse with a machine than with the hand shears. If the cutter is held down too far on one side a furrow is plowed through the sheep's skin. Some shearers who are not careful when performing this work cut off the ends of the teats of ewes, which spoils them for

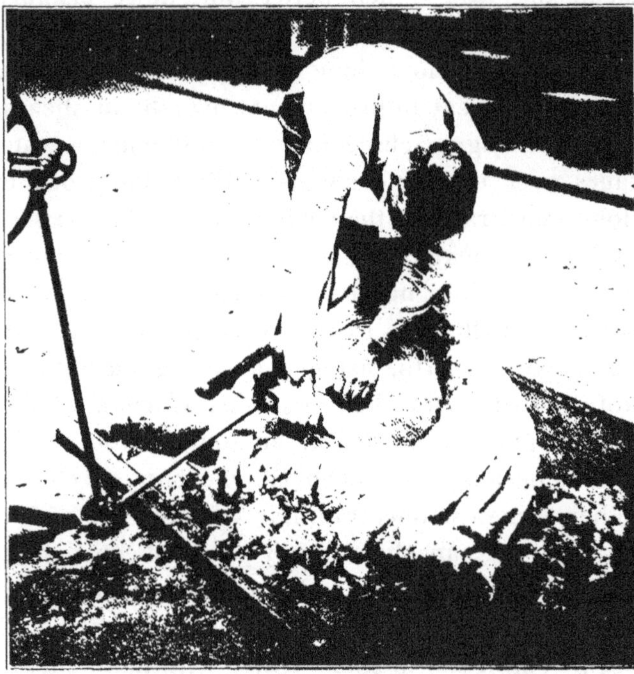

PLATE 32. Shearing sheep with a shearing machine at the University of Wisconsin.

nursing lambs. Others cut off the end of the vagina, which, it is claimed by some authorities, stops them from further breeding. Such men as these should certainly not be allowed to shear sheep.

In older countries shearers tie up all four legs of the sheep to prevent it from struggling. This old-fashioned way, however, should not be practiced in America. A sheep, if properly held, cannot do a great deal of struggling. Just how to hold the sheep in the many different positions necessary while shearing it could hardly be fully explained, but must be learned through actual practice. The best way for the beginner to learn how to hold and shear sheep is to watch an expert shear a few sheep. It may be stated, however, that in every position the sheep must be held so as to draw the skin tight where the shearer is working. The sheep should also always be held in the most comfortable position instead of in the cramped positions in which some shearers hold sheep. One of the positions in which the sheep is held while being sheared is shown in the accompanying illustration.

TYING UP THE FLEECE.

The fleeces should be neatly tied up in order to make them look attractive to the buyer. The side of the fleece which was next to the sheep's skin should be placed on the outside when the fleece is tied up, in such a way that no parts of the former exterior of the fleece when on the sheep are seen in the bundle. This can be done very easily by a good shearer, as he should be able to take off a fleece from a sheep all in one piece, like an overcoat, with the exception, perhaps, of the belly piece. Regular wool twine should be used in tying up the wool. Binder twine or other sharp cord should never be used, as small bits of fiber get into the wool and must be picked out by hand since they do not take dyes. Therefore manufacturers object seriously to the use of such twine, and make a reduction in the price of the wool if it is used. All filthy parts on the fleece, if there should be any at all, should be separated at the time the fleece is tied up and never tied up with the fleece, for a man can fool a buyer but once.

Since the first publication of this work, however, a new kind of wool twine has been made which fills all requirements from the standpoint of the woolen manufacturer, namely, the paper twine. This new twine, which can be bought cheaply, is smooth and never tangles up with the fibers of the wool. As wool buyers pay more per pound for fleeces that are free from the sisals, which cannot be left in the wool, this kind of twine is highly recommended and should be used wherever sheep are sheared.

A wool buyer once told the writer about a man from whom he had bought very heavy fleeces of wool. On closer examination he found that the fleeces had been sprinkled with sand at the time of tying them up, to make them heavier in weight. Another man had tied up a sheep's skin in a fleece. Still others had turned their sheep out during a

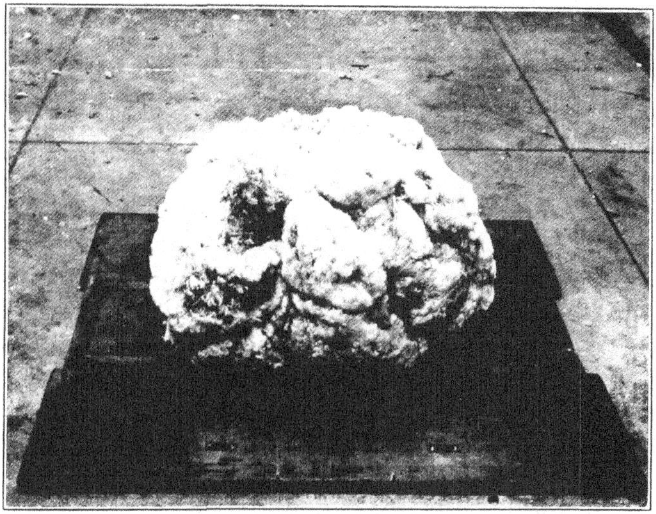

PLATE 33. An unusually heavy fleece, weighing 17.25 pounds, taken from a Shropshire ram at the University of Wisconsin.

rain in order to increase the weight of wool. All such tricks as these are soon disclosed, and in the future work strongly against the men who perform them. Therefore, brother sheepmen, always be honest and do not be guilty of such trickery, for you will find that honesty is always the best policy.

A wool box may be used in tying up the fleeces, the use of which will add greatly to their attractiveness. The accompanying illustration shows a well tied fleece, lying on the wool box by means of which it was tied. However, wool buyers prefer to have the fleeces tied up neatly without the use of the wool box, as less twine is then used. If one is careful in removing the fleece from the sheep a fleece may be tied up in a satisfactory manner without the use of the wool box.

SHEARING EWES BEFORE OR AFTER LAMBING.

When ewes have been bred late in the fall, which of course, brings them to lamb late in the spring, they can be sheared before lambing. Shearing the ewes before lambing has the following advantages: Ewes sheared before coming in keep much cleaner at the rear than those with their wool on. There is also no danger of lambs biting off wool from their mothers and swallowing it, which will cause balls of wool to form in their intestines, thus stopping up the bowels and killing the lambs. When the ewes are shorn lambs will find their mother's teats more easily, and the time taken to trim the wool away around the udder is saved. Another point in favor of shearing before lambing is the fact that ewes with their coats on often remain outdoors during rains or severe cold, and their lambs naturally stay at their side. The old sheep, being well protected by their fleeces, do not mind the rain or the cold, but the young lamb with its short wool gets chilled or wet to the skin and catches cold, this often bringing on pneumonia and finally resulting in the death of the lamb. On the other hand, if the old sheep have been sheared at this time and the barn doors are left open for them, they will run to the barn and seek shelter just as soon as it turns cold or begins to rain, thereby protecting not only themselves but also their lambs. Some of our best sheep breeders favor shearing before lambing, and keep up this practice each year. Of course, these men do their shearing themselves and in the most careful manner.

When ewes are sheared before lambing, only the most competent and careful shearers should ever perform the work, and even such men must use extreme care and patience to make sure that none of the ewes heavy with lamb are injured, resulting in abortion. Therefore, unless the most competent and painstaking shearers can be secured, in spite of the advantages of shearing before lambing, the writer would in general advise that ewes lamb before being sheared. However, when ewes are due to lamb late in the season it may be best to shear them before they lamb.

DIPPING A NECESSITY.

At least once a year the flock should be dipped in order to rid it from ticks and also from lice, if the latter should be present. The best time to dip is shortly after shearing. A nice, warm, sunshiny day should be selected for this work, and it should preferably be done in the morning so as to give the sheep a chance to dry out again before night. Any one of the many recommended coal tar dips may be used. Dipping the flock is strongly advised not only for the purpose of killing ticks and lice but also in order to promote the health of the skin and to further the growth of the wool. For this reason many sheep breeders dip each year, in spite of the fact that they know their flocks are free from vermin. Many even dip twice a year, in spring and in fall, because they realize the benefit derived therefrom.

In case a flockmaster does not find time to dip his whole flock because of the rush of other farm work, he ought at least dip the lambs in the spring. As a rule not many flocks are entirely free from ticks. If the old sheep have been sheared clean and no patches of wool are left on them ticks will move off from them and find new homes and shelter on the lambs, which have more wool on them at this time than the old sheep that have been sheared. Eight to ten days after shearing all the ticks will have moved off from the old sheep onto the lambs, and the lambs should be dipped to destroy them. It is preferable, however, to dip the entire flock if possible.

In dipping the sheep it is not necessary for the head of the sheep to get into the dip, as the ticks or lice will hardly ever be found here, since the sheep can rub and scratch its head easily, thus keeping these pests off from this part. Furthermore, it is not the best thing for a sheep to get the dip into its mouth, eyes, and ears. However, all other parts of the body up to the head, should be kept in the dip not less than one minute. The dip will be more effective if the solution is lukewarm, and the sheep will not then be chilled when taking a bath in it.

The cut on page 88 shows the pen into which sheep are driven when they are to be dipped, the dipping vat, and the draining pen, where the sheep remain until they have nicely drained. The vat is made of galvanized iron, and is movable, so that after all the sheep are dipped, the vat can be stored away in the draining pen, where it will be well protected and will therefore last for many years. The size of the vat necessary depends on the size of the flock kept on the farm. The draining pen is so arranged that all the dip which runs off the sheep while they are dripping runs back into the vat.

The writer does not understand why dipping is neglected by some sheep owners. It is impossible for sheep to make any progress when they are covered with ticks and lice which annoy them day and night. When sheep are infested with these pests they have no rest at all. They are kept busy biting their wool and scratching continuously and seeking every sharp corner or post to rub against in fighting the insects.

It is difficult to estimate how much feed is wasted and how much flesh is lost when ticks or lice are present in a flock. It is certain, however, that a great portion of the feed consumed by the sheep helps to support these pests. They suck much blood out of the sheep, and this blood which the sheep needs for its maintenance must be restored through the feed, which should be used by the sheep for its growth and development. Therefore it is very unwise to let sheep suffer from such pests through failure to dip them at least once a year.

TRIMMING THE FEET

It is most essential that sheep have their feet taken care of just as well as any other part of their bodies. It is necessary to attend to their feet, first, to prevent foot rot, and second, to avoid crooked and broken-down pasterns. There is some difference in the amount of care necessary for the various breeds of sheep. In general, the feet of sheep which produce the finest grade of wool need

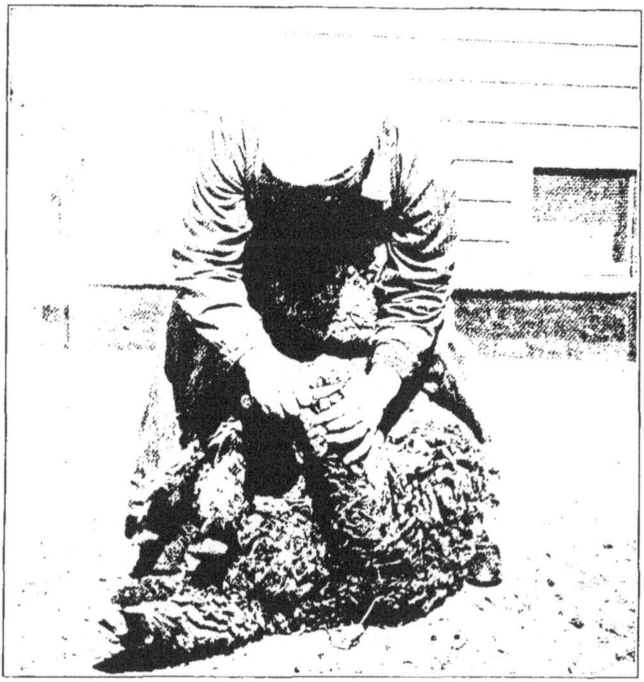

PLATE 34. Trimming the hoofs of a sheep with a jack-knife.

most attention. The hoof of the Merino, which has the finest wool, grows much more rapidly than that of other breeds, and the feet of Southdowns, the breed next finest in wool, also need more attention than do the Oxfords, Cheviots, or long wool breeds, which have the coarser fleeces. However, any breed of sheep ought to have its feet trimmed at least twice a year, in spring and fall. Fine wool breeds, as mentioned before, should be given attention in this respect oftener than twice a year. When sheep are neglected with regard to this matter the outside horny part of the hoof grows over the sole. A hollow space is thus left between hoof and sole in which dirt collects, and this finally begins to make the foot sore, with the result that foot rot sets in.

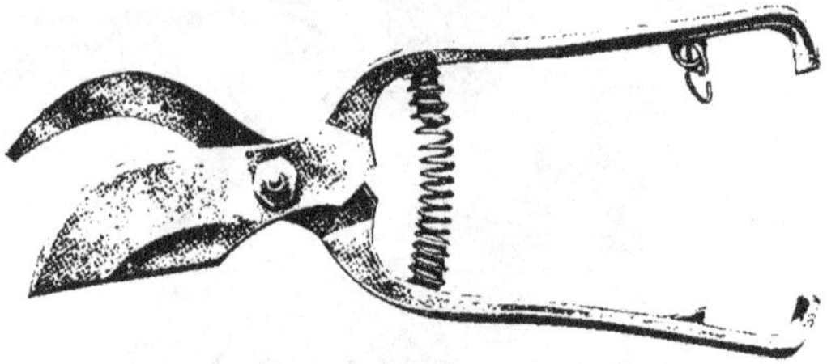

PLATE 35. Pruning knife, or clippers, used in removing the largest portions of the surplus hoof.

As has been mentioned, the second danger is in crooked and broken-down pasterns. Many good sheep have been disregarded in the show ring on account of crooked feet and broken-down pasterns, due to neglect of the shepherd in not trimming their feet at the proper time. Foot trimming is a phase of sheep husbandry that requires the flockmaster's attention just the same as feeding and shearing.

In the spring after shearing is the best time to trim the feet of the flock. In order to do this work quickly it is well to turn the sheep out on damp ground for several hours, which will clean their hoofs and make the horny part soft so that it will cut easily. A clipper, also called a pruning knife, such as is shown in the illustration, may be used to remove the largest portion of the surplus hoof, and a sharp jack-knife to finish it. If the feet are properly softened a jack-knife may do all the work satisfactorily. The hoof should be cut down so as to make it level with the sole of the foot. In some cases one side will need a little more cutting than the other in order to make the foot stand straight when placed on the ground. A. O. Fox, one of the oldest and foremost sheep breeders in Wisconsin, once said to the writer: "A shepherd who does not take care of the feet of his flock is just as dangerous as the one who does not feed his flock properly," and this is certainly true.

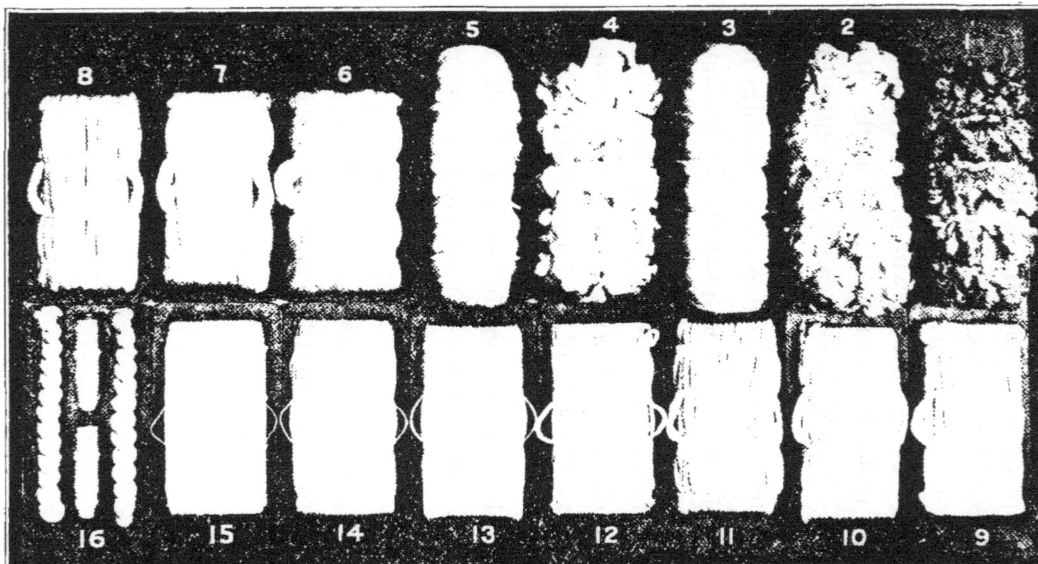

PLATE 36. The different processes required to manufacture the fleece into yarn. No. 1, the fleece; No. 2, scoured; No. 3, card sliver; No. 4 noils; No. 5, top; Nos. 6-15, drawing slivers; No. 16, yarn. Courtesy National Wool Warehouse & Storage Co., Chicago, Ill.

CHAPTER VI.

PREVENTION AND TREATMENT OF PARASITES.

The flockmaster has little work with his sheep in the summer when they are on pasture, aside from keeping them free from parasites. These insects have caused the loss of thousands of lambs and sheep and have, in some cases, discouraged the flockowners so thoroughly that they have dropped out of the sheep business. Among these parasites the stomach worm is perhaps the one that has done the most damage to sheep husbandry. On land where rotation of crops is not practiced and old meadow pastures that cannot be tilled are used continuously during many years for pasturing sheep, the infection with parasites is much greater than on land where the rotation plan is followed and sheep are changed to new, fresh ground each year. The danger of stomach worms is not nearly so great in winter as in summer, and the months of July, August, and September are the most serious times for the flockowner. The writer has known, nevertheless, of a few instances where sheep have died in winter and early spring from infection with these pests.

SYMPTOMS OF STOMACH WORMS.

A person who is familiar with the subject of sheep husbandry can easily detect any member in the flock that is infested with stomach worms. The sheep so infested usually hangs back from the rest of the flock, walks somewhat stiff, and shows loss of flesh. Its wool becomes harsh and appears dry and in many cases the sheep will scour. The sheep looks weak and dull and lets its head hang low, and it often happens that a soft kind of swelling forms under the lower jaw during the day time and disappears again by the next morning. In this condition sheep eat a great deal of earth wherever they find it and drink more water than usual. Some of them withstand these worms for a long time, while others die within two weeks to ten days or even a shorter period from the time they first show symptoms of the disease. Many sheep may die in a flock, and yet the owner will have no clue as to the cause of their death. In order to make sure that a sheep which shows any of the foregoing symptoms is suffering from worms, pull down its lower eyelid and note the color of the mucous membrane, or inside lining, of the eyelid. It should be of a pink color, showing an abundance of blood. If, however, it is of a pale, yellowish color and the skin on the side of the sheep also appears pale when the wool is parted, the owner may invariably be certain that stomach worms are at work in the sheep. This pale condition is due to the fact that these worms suck all the blood out of the animal, and it will finally die because of this loss of blood. When lambs which are badly infested with these worms are killed they have been found to have scarcely any blood left in them.

Stomach worms are only found in the fourth stomach of the sheep. When this stomach is carefully opened a dark brown fluid will be observed, which contains thousands of little worms of a reddish color, about three-fourths of an inch or an inch long and as thick as a hair. This mass of worms is responsible for the death of the lamb. It may be in place to repeat here that older sheep are not subject to stomach worms as commonly as are lambs, but the writer wishes it clearly understood that older sheep are not entirely exempt from these pests. As far as is known these worms get their start in the body of the older sheep and pass out in the droppings. It is thought that when these worms leave the sheep they are loaded with eggs which soon hatch. The young worms do not stay down on the ground but seek a temporary abode on the stems and leaves of grass and are thus swallowed by sheep grazing thereon. These worms are perhaps thickest around the shade trees in pastures, where sheep spend most of their time during the hottest hours of the summer day. Most of the droppings of the ewes are found here and consequently the freshest and nicest grass grows in this place. The innocent lambs get up from their shady resting place, begin nibbling on this fresh-looking grass, eat grass and worms together, and the worms find their natural homes in the lambs' stomachs and begin the work of destruction at once. It is peculiar that older sheep possess a certain instinct which keeps them from eating very much near shade trees but leads them off for a distance, just as if they realized the danger at hand. The lambs, like other young animals, are easily caught in the trap, and thus are infested with the worms more than the older sheep. The older sheep also seem to possess more power to resist the attacks of stomach worms. Experiments carried on at the experiment stations have clearly demonstrated that lambs get these parasites on pasture. At the Ohio Experiment Station lambs that were fed all summer in a barn were kept free from parasites, while others that were turned out to pasture were badly infested.

THE PREVENTION OF STOMACH WORMS.

It is far easier to prevent infection with stomach worms than it is to destroy the worms when the sheep have become infested with them. Nothing can be more highly recommended for the prevention of stomach worms in sheep than the frequent change of pasture, for sheep become infested with these pests only by swallowing the worms while grazing. If possible sheep should be changed to fresh, clean pasture every two to three weeks during June, July, August, and September, for during warm weather otherwise clean pastures may become infested in even less time by sheep grazing thereon. Fields on which no sheep or goats have grazed for a year, and plots which have been plowed and cultivated since sheep grazed on them are practically free from infection. Old blue grass pastures are especially to be avoided. It is thus clear that annual pastures, such as rape, furnish clean pasture for the flock. In the warmer sections it is necessary to begin changing to fresh pasture earlier in the spring and to change more frequently in the summer. This method requires several separate, clean pasture lots, but flockmasters who have followed this method have had little trouble with parasites.

In some cases it is impossible for the flockmaster to change pastures as frequently as has been recommended above. For such instances it is to be hoped that some remedy may be found which will be a sure preventative of stomach worms. During the last few years some medicated stock salts have been placed on the market which the manufacturers claim will prevent and destroy all parasites in sheep, but at this time the writer is unable to state whether these products will do the work satisfactorily or not. Some breeders claim that feeding tobacco prevents parasites. Others recommend the use of turpentine and wood ashes, mixed with salt.

Sheep should never be allowed to drink stagnant water from old ponds or mud holes in which all sorts of insects live. When sheep are allowed to drink such stagnant water, covered with a green scum, they are liable to become infested with parasites and also contract many diseases such as anthrax and others nearly as serious. The writer wishes to again impress upon flockmasters the great danger of allowing their sheep to drink such stagnant water. Fresh, pure water should be provided for the sheep every day of the year, and as much of it as they want. The idea so commonly held that sheep do not need water is entirely wrong. Sheep should always have access to fresh, pure water, since they need it just as much as any other farm animal.

TREATMENT FOR STOMACH WORMS.

A number of remedies can be recommended which have proved satisfactory for destroying stomach worms. Gasoline, turpentine, benzine, and others are excellent for this purpose, and will also destroy tape worms in sheep. Among these remedies gasoline is the writer's favorite, for in his experience this has given the best results.

The unfortunate lambs or sheep that are to undergo this treatment should be separated from the rest of the flock in the evening and be shut off in a barnyard or perhaps a stable, where they cannot get anything to eat or drink over night. In the morning the stomachs will be fairly empty and this will render it possible for the dose to enter quickly into the fourth stomach of the sheep, where the worms are located. The sheep will therefore now be ready for the first dose.

SIZE OF DOSE.

When either gasoline, turpentine, or benzine is used, the size of the dose is practically the same. The dose *for lambs* is as follows:

5 ounces of cow's whole milk.
1¼ tablespoonful of gasoline.
1 tablespoonful of raw linseed oil.

This dose, which is to be mixed up separately for each lamb, should be well shaken in a small-necked bottle like that in Plate 37 and given to the lamb. For older sheep the dose of gasoline, turpentine, or benzine is from one and one-half tablespoonfuls to two tablespoons (not teaspoonfuls) according to the size of the sheep, while the amount of milk and of linseed oil is the same. This treatment, when repeated for each animal for three successive mornings, will certainly, if handled right, be a cure for stomach worms. Of course, each time the sheep must have been deprived of all food over night. The dose may be given every alternate day in case the lambs have become very weak before the trouble was noticed. Some authorities recommend that another single dose of the mixture be given ten days after the third dose. In former years the writer used only the milk and gasoline for dosing, but in later years he has also added linseed oil, for the reason that lambs take this mixture more easily and do not mind the strength of the gasoline so much when it passes through the mouth and throat. This linseed oil also helps to carry off the worms that are killed, but does not weaken the dose in any way.

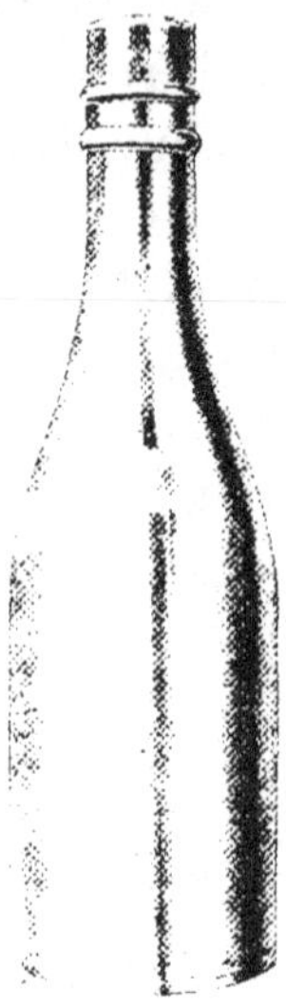

PLATE 37. Drenching bottle.

DRENCHING SHEEP.

Great precautions must be taken when administering medicine to sheep so as not to strangle them, as even some older sheepmen have choked lambs by drenching them. Giving medicine to sheep is not a serious job, however, if enough care is exercised. In administering medicine place the lambs to be treated in a narrow space so that they may be caught without chasing, catch one, and back it into a corner. If the sheep is small enough, straddle it, otherwise stand on its right side as is shown in the accompanying illustration. Now place your left hand on its jaw with the thumb of the left hand in its mouth on the tongue and between the front and back teeth, opening the mouth so that the neck of the bottle may be placed on its tongue. Be careful not to hold its head up too high, for in this unnatural position it may choke. Pour the contents of the bottle slowly down

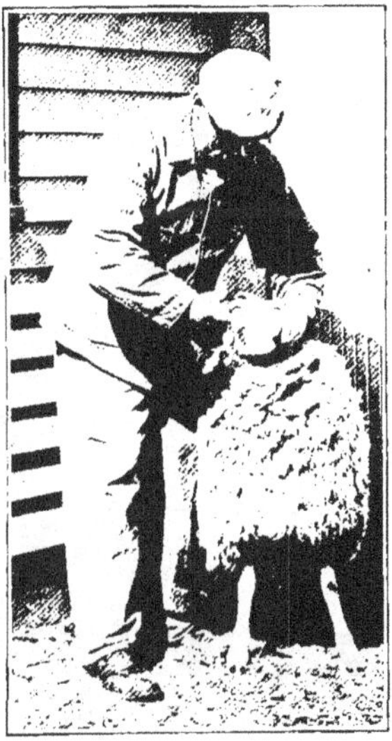

PLATE 38. The manner in which a large sheep is drenched.

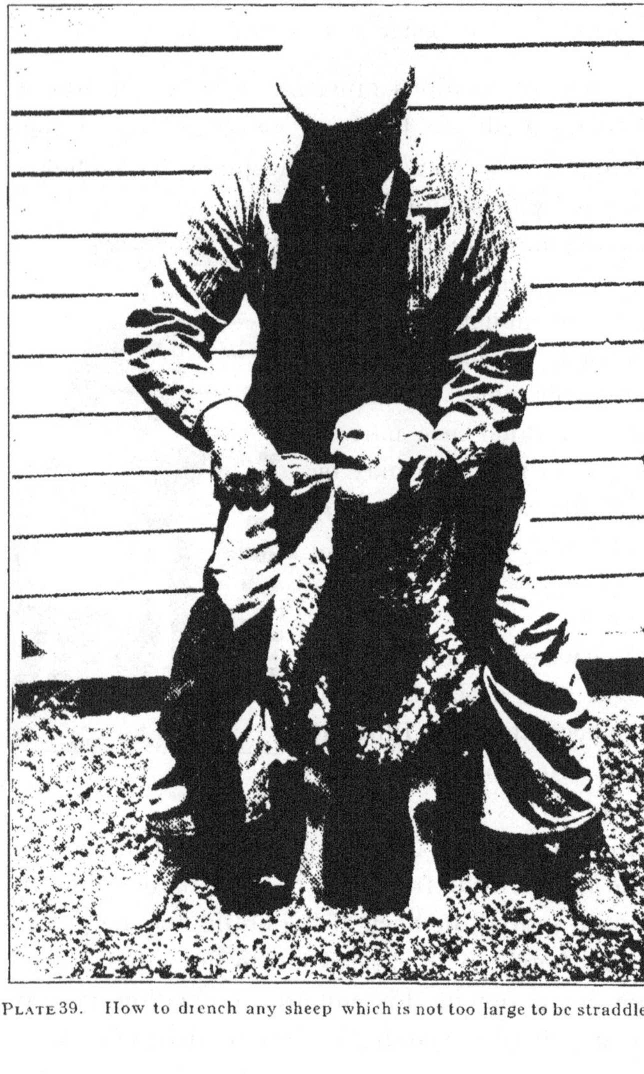

PLATE 39. How to drench any sheep which is not too large to be straddled.

its throat, perhaps one-third or one-half of it at one time. Wait for a minute, then give some more until all is taken. At least one or two pauses should be made in order that a part of the dose may not enter the lungs and prove fatal to the sheep. The fingers of the left hand by which the lamb's head is held should be left free, and the under jaw should not be held tight up against the upper jaw, which would, of course, prevent the lamb from swallowing, and consequently the medicine would run down into its lungs and kill the lamb instantly. An incorrect method of holding lambs when drenching has killed many of them. Some shepherds practice setting the sheep on its rump with its head held high, but in the author's experience this has not been found advisable. When the sheep's head is held too high it cannot swallow very well and the dose runs down its windpipe into its lungs. This method of holding the sheep should be followed not alone when sheep are drenched to kill parasites but in all cases where it is necessary for medicine to be given. Be very particular to keep the fingers of your left hand off from the under jaw while the medicine is being given, and all will be well. Shortly after dosing the lambs with gasoline or other remedies they may again be turned out on grass each day.

SHEEP WITH GRUB IN THE HEAD.

Another evil to be feared in sheep husbandry is grub in the head of sheep. Experienced sheepmen generally admit that sheep which are grazing in brush and woodland are in greater danger of being troubled with these grubs than sheep which are feeding on clear pastures.

In the hot summer weather while the sheep is resting beside bushes and shady trees chewing its cud or perhaps sleeping, a big fly lights on its nose. Generally a little fluid, not at all harmful, is running from the nostrils of the sheep. This fly settles down on the nostrils and at times will even crawl up into the sheep's nose in order to feed on this fluid. In the meantime it also deposits some eggs or perhaps young worms, which the sheep in breathing draws up into its head between the eyes where there are cavities in the nasal passages. The eggs hatch, or the worms develop into large-sized grubs, which look like those commonly found under rotten stumps or plowed sod ground. The only difference is that the grubs found in the head of sheep, when full grown, are not quite half the size of those seen in the field or under stumps. In some instances as many as eleven of such grubs of different sizes and ages have been found in a single sheep that had died with grub in the head.

When a sheep has grub in the head it lets its head hang down to the ground, grinds its teeth frequently, turns its head to one side, then to the other, and then back towards its shoulders, and often walks around in a circle. A green liquid may run out of its nose, and of course it has also lost its appetite. When sheep become infested with grub in the head it is a very fatal matter, as no reliable cure for it has as yet been found.

Some years ago the writer took a trip to Europe to study sheep husbandry on that continent. He there met some of the oldest shepherds, who had spent their whole lives in herding and caring for sheep and had therefore gained much practical experience. These shepherds claimed that some sheep could be saved by letting a little snuff tobacco thoroughly mixed with linseed oil run into the sheep's nostrils. By holding the sheep's head high when the mixture was poured into the nostrils it would find its way to the place where the grubs were lodged. The grubs would be disturbed by this snuff and the sheep would begin to sneeze and thus force the grubs out of the head. This may be a good remedy, and those sheepmen who are troubled with this pest might give it a trial, but the author has had no occasion to test it as he has always succeeded in preventing grub in the head by the method which follows.

PREVENTION.

This disease in sheep can be avoided by doing a little extra work. If no other time is suitable for this purpose it can be done in the evening after supper when the other chores are completed, as the

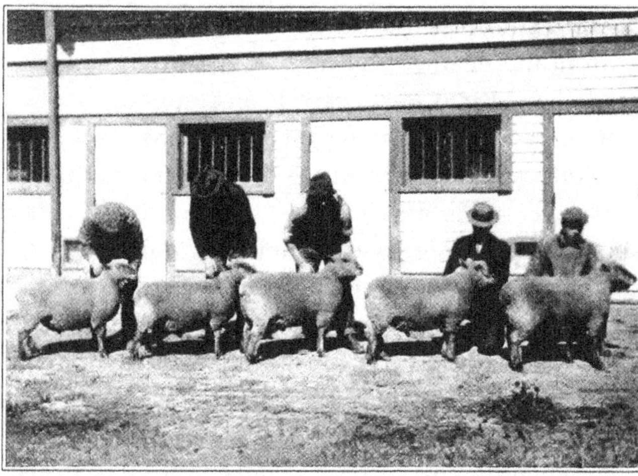

PLATE 40. Five purebred Southdown yearling wethers fitted by the University of Wisconsin for the 1915 International show which was not held because of the prevalence of the foot and mouth disease

days are longest in fly time, which is in summer. It is an old saying that where there is a will there is a way, and so it is here. A man who has a small flock can probably take the time, say every two or three weeks, to smear some pine tar on the noses of the sheep. Even if the sheep eat a little of it, it will not harm them, on the contrary, it is good for them. The tar will keep the flies away from the sheeps' noses, and in fact away from any place where it is present, for flies despise pine tar.

It is important to see to it that sheep have free access to salt at all times of the year, whether they are in the barn or on pasture. This salt, however, should be placed in a salt box and not thrown on the ground, as some careless flockowners do. In summer smear the bottom and sides of the salt trough with a heavy coat of pine tar, and then sprinkle the salt on top of it. In licking up the salt sheep cannot avoid getting some tar on their noses, and herein lies the whole secret of this method of preventing grubs. The flies will now no longer bother their noses. This is a simple but effective method of preventing grub in the head Rock salt, of course, can not be used for this purpose, but common salt is now so cheap that it hardly pays to use the rock salt anyway.

In Canada the writer has seen still another method practiced. A log is selected and holes bored into it with an auger, each hole being wide and deep enough so that the sheep can get its nose into it nearly up to the eyes. These holes are about three feet apart. They are smeared on the inside with a heavy coat of pine tar and the holes are filled up with salt. In this manner the sheep get even more tar on their noses than they will in eating salt from the trough. Either of these methods is a good and simple way to keep sheep free from grub in the head.

BLOAT IN SHEEP.

Sheep, as a rule, are very greedy. When turned on some new pasture, such as clover, alfalfa, or rape, they eat too fast and too much and consequently bloat. Any one of these forages will bloat sheep very quickly when the crop is too young, fresh, and juicy. The weather conditions also have something to do with this. Even if sheep have been grazing on clover or alfalfa fields without any symptoms of bloating for some time, all danger is not yet over. Some night a heavy rain or thunderstorm may sweep over the country, and the next day be very warm and sultry, indicating more rain to follow. On such a day as this, no matter how safe your sheep have been on this same field before, something is very likely to happen. There is not so much danger in the forenoon as in the afternoon, especially late in the afternoon towards sunset and evening. The moisture in the ground from a previous rain seems to have an effect on the clover, and the latter then seems to form more gas when in the sheep's stomach, resulting in bloat. Many shepherds have been in great anxiety when they came to their flock and found five or six sheep lying dead before them, bloated as big as barrels, and others suffering from bloat.

Sheep that have eaten large quantities of clover, rape, or alfalfa and have become bloated, are in terrible distress. The gas rising from fermentation causes the first stomach to distend to its utmost capacity. This stomach on account of its abnormal size presses upon the lungs, and consequently interferes with the respiration, sometimes stopping it entirely, in which case death follows, or the stomach may even burst from the pressure.

REMEDY FOR BLOAT.

Trocars and knives have been used in tapping the bloated sheep to let the gas escape from the stomach. The writer must confess that he never had any success with either of the two, perhaps due to his own fault in operation. But he takes pride in giving to his readers a remedy, still unknown to many and not yet published elsewhere. When the sheep that is bloated is not found altogether too late, and the overloaded stomach has not been pressing too heavily upon the lungs or has not burst, the sheep can be saved. Quickly find a pail, run to the first cow you see that is giving milk, draw out from a pint to a quart of it, come back to the sheep as quickly as possible, and give about a

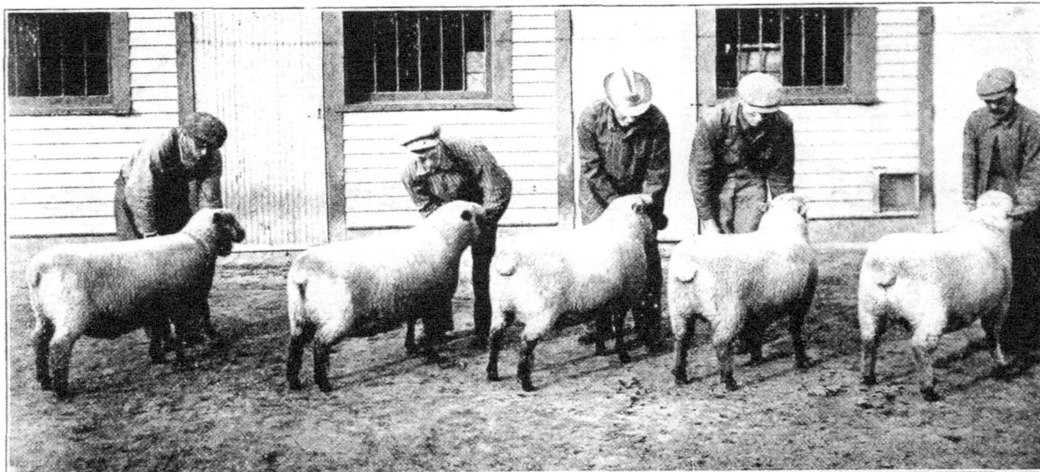

PLATE 41. First prize pen of five grade Shropshire yearling wethers at the International, 1913. Shown by the University of Wisconsin.

half pint of the warm milk to the sheep by means of the drenching bottle. If it does not stop groaning and stretching in a short time give it another half pint of milk. Soon after this you will see the animal draw in its bulged-out sides and begin to look smaller, and after a little it will have regained its natural form. The writer has saved many bloated sheep in this way. Remember that the milk must be warm from the cow's udder. Cold milk does not absorb the gas as the warm milk does. Give the milk as warm as possible, and be careful not to choke the sheep when dosing it in this bloated condition.

SOME COMMON MEDICINES HELPFUL TO THE FLOCK-MASTER.

It is generally conceded that if a sheep once gets sick not much can be done to save it. The writer, however, is not exactly of this opinion. True enough, if a sheep has pneumonia and its lungs are badly affected death is generally the result. There are other diseases which baffle even the knowledge and control of veterinarians. In many instances, however, the shepherd can himself treat the sick sheep in lighter cases. For instance, if a sheep suffers from constipation this trouble can be removed by giving the sheep one or perhaps two doses of epsom salts. The dose for an older sheep is from four to five ounces and for a lamb somewhat less. This salt is dissolved in warm water and given in a drench. If the bowels do not move in from five to six hours a second dose may be given, adding a little castor oil to it. In some bad cases an injection of warm water with a little soap in it is helpful in getting the bowels to move. A dose of epsom salts is also beneficial for a sheep that has contracted a bad cold.

Little lambs sometimes become constipated from their mother's milk, in which cases one-half to one teaspoonful of castor oil given the youngster once or twice will remedy the trouble.

COLIC, OR "STRETCHES."

This trouble is caused by the sheep eating frozen roots, corn silage that contains a great amount of acid or which has been frozen a little, or any other food that chills the stomach of the sheep. The symptoms of colic or so-called stretches in sheep are: stretching the body much longer than it really is; turning over on one side, then on the other; lying down for a few minutes, and then getting up again; stretching the body out again so that the sheep appears to be sway-backed.

A tablespoonful of sweet spirits of nitre given in a little water will relieve the sheep of its pains. Sometimes a second dose has to be given if the sheep is not relieved of its distress by the first dose.

WETHERS WITH SORE SHEATHS.

Wethers often become sore at the end of their sheath and penis. Such cases should be treated by injections of permanganate of potash solution with a small syringe, repeating a number of times and using one-half teaspoonful of permanganate of potash to a quart of warm water. After each injection a little iodoform should be applied to the sore on the end of the sheath.

MAGGOTS IN MIDSUMMER AND FLY TIME.

Another pest that needs the shepherd's close attention during the hot weather and fly time is the maggot. These maggots have caused great loss to the flockowner and a most terrible death to the poor, innocent sheep that are infested. It is terrible to think of a harmless sheep being eaten alive by hundreds of thousands of these maggots, which steadily gnaw and feed on its body until finally the animal succumbs. Yet this unhappy lot has befallen many sheep. You may ask whether it is possible for a person to be so cruel as to let his sheep be eaten alive. It is true enough, but why and how is this done? Simply because some people have not yet learned what particular precautions must be taken at certain times of the season in order to prevent this evil, or they are altogether too careless in managing their flocks. For instance a man

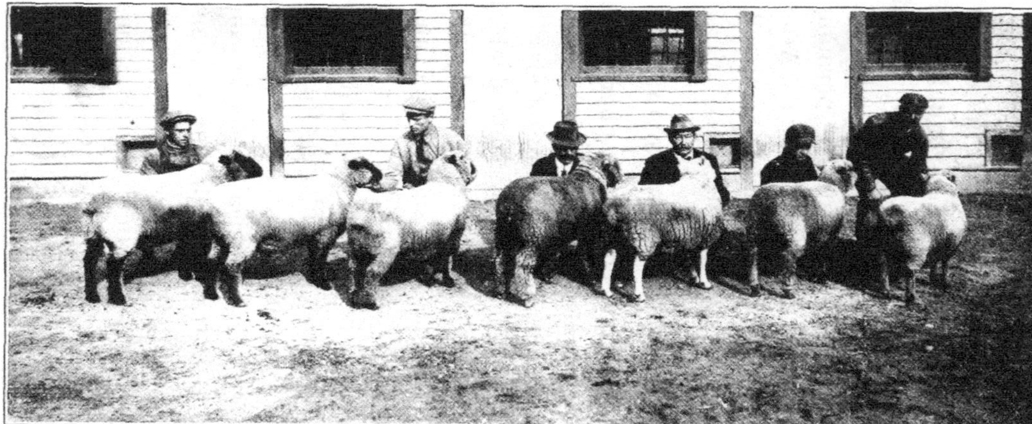

PLATE 42. A group of different breeds of yearling wethers which were prepared by the University of Wisconsin for the 1914 International show, which was not held on account of the prevalence of the foot and mouth disease.

starts in sheep husbandry, is in earnest about it, and wants to do the best he can. The first summer he keeps sheep may be a very favorable one and everything may run smoothly throughout the season. The next year the season may be much different, but he fears nothing because he had no trouble whatever the first year. Some day he will find a stumbling block in his way, which he has not seen or heard of up to this time. He may find one or two of his sheep lying dead in the pasture. He makes an examination, and behold, what meets his eye? Thousands and thousands of little white maggots are having a feast on the dead sheep. He now begins to wonder what could have been the trouble with his sheep. It is a puzzle to him whether these maggots got on to the sheep after it had died, or whether they got on while it was still alive and then killed it. Only a few years ago a farmer came to this Station and asked for information concerning the cause of the death of thirteen head of sheep, which he thought were eaten up by worms. The writer asked the question: "Where were the worms that killed your sheep, inside the sheep's body or on the outside?" The farmer replied that many little white worms, about half an inch long, were seen on the outside of the sheep. Evidently maggots were at work on his flock and he did not know it, as he stated that he had never heard of maggots killing sheep.

CAUSE OF MAGGOTS.

Maggots on sheep are caused by blow-flies. Female sheep are more apt to have maggots than male sheep, although males also occasionally become infested. Sheep sometimes get filthy on their bodies, especially at the rear, caused either by their scouring, or in the case of females by the spattering of the urine on the wool. The so-called blow-fly comes along, feeds on this filth, and meanwhile lays eggs there. These eggs hatch, forming tiny worm-like larvae, which grow fast, and burrow into the flesh of the sheep. In a couple of days a large patch of full grown maggots are present on the sheep, more eggs are laid and hatch, and in the course of three or four days maggots are there by the thousands. On account of the rapid increase in number these maggots move forward and spread over the body of the sheep, and after six or seven days the sheep dies a lingering death.

PREVENTION.

In hot weather and fly time the conscientious shepherd makes it a point to inspect his flock in the pasture at least once a day. If he should notice any filthy portions of wool on any member in the flock he will quickly get a pair of shears and cut them off. He also will get a solution of some coal tar sheep dip, mixed in the proportions of one part of dip to seventy-five parts of water, and cleanse the filthy portions thoroughly. It may be added here that if no dip is left over after sheep dipping time is past some more ought to be secured for use during the summer. The odor left on the sheep by this solution will keep the flies away for quite a long period. When proper attention is given the sheep, maggots will not find their way onto any members of the flock.

TREATMENT OF MAGGOTS.

When sheep are already infested with maggots the same treatment should be used as is used to prevent maggots. The wool must be cut away as close to the skin as possible and as far as these miserable pests are lodged. The infested portion should then be washed with a solution of dip consisting of one part of dip to fifty of water. As the maggots are unable to withstand the odor of the dip they will then fall to the ground. Sometimes they will already have made large holes in the body of the sheep, in which case care must be taken to cleanse these thoroughly and remove all maggots. It is a good plan to smear some pine tar in these holes after all the maggots have been cleaned out.

Many sheepmen use turpentine to kill maggots. The writer, however, does not favor its use for the reason that it is too strong and sharp and bites the skin of the sheep, making it very raw and causing the animal severe pain. A solution of Zenoleum or Creso dip are mild on the skin, are disinfectants, and at the same time have a healing effect.

CHAPTER VII.

SUMMER FEEDING AND CARE.

After the winter and early spring work is all done, the flock is put out on pasture to enjoy the young, juicy grass. The shepherd should be careful to provide pure, fresh water, salt, and shade for the sheep on pasture, in order that the flock may thrive properly. At this time he is relieved more or less from the restless hours and worry of lambing, shearing, and feet trimming, and is enjoying a little rest. He must now, however, begin to think about work that may be done in the field to provide some kind of forage to help him out with his flock at the time when pastures are generally short and scanty on account of the dry weather of midsummer. He must also bear in mind that when the time comes to wean lambs he should have a fresh piece of pasture for them away from the older sheep. In some cases the lambs may be grazed on a field from which the first crop of hay has been taken. Even if such a pasture is available a piece of rape should be sown in the spring early enough to be ripe July 25 to August 10, the usual time for weaning lambs, for rape is an excellent fodder for lambs. Indeed rape has

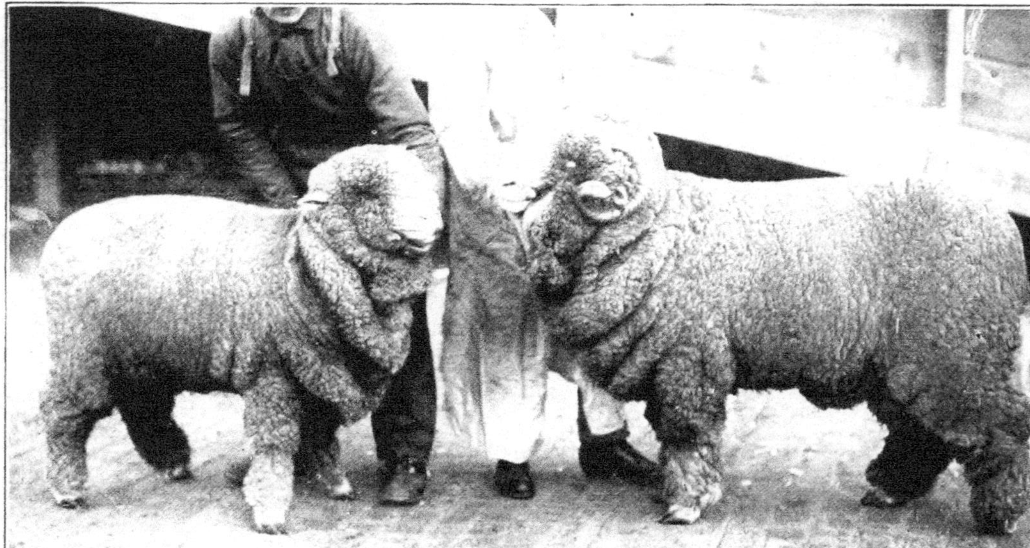

PLATE 13. Champion Rambouillet ram and ewe at the International, 1910, shown by F. S. King Bros., Wyoming.

an unusual value for feeding all classes of sheep, and a great amount of feed can be obtained from an acre. It may be sown broadcast, or it may be drilled in. If time permits, it is far better to sow it in rows thirty inches apart, as much more feed can then be grown on an acre and the crop can also be cultivated, thus holding the weeds in check. Sheep will then waste but little of the rape when turned into it, as they will walk between the rows and eat on both sides.

Roots, such as rutabagas and turnips, should also be sown for late fall and winter feeding. Good roots are just as well liked by sheep in the winter time as cake and pie are liked by man. They should be kept in a well-ventilated cellar where they will not freeze or rot. Cabbage is an excellent feed for all classes of sheep, but is usually too expensive to feed extensively. However, where large fields of cabbage are grown for the market, sheep can well be fed the leaves and unsalable heads which are left after the crop is harvested.

SUGAR BEETS AND MANGELS A DANGEROUS FEED FOR RAMS AND WETHERS.

For many years sheep breeders in this country as well as in England have been aware of the fact that sugar beets and mangels are dangerous for ram and wether feeding. Trials covering five years at the Iowa Experiment Station have shown this to be true. The writer in his earlier years, not having had as much experience as he should have had, learned costly lessons by feeding these roots to rams and wethers and consequently losing a number of good, high-priced animals. Mangels and sugar beets contain some alkali substances which affect the kidneys and form gravel stones in the kidneys and bladder, stopping up the passage of the urinary canal. When this passage is blocked, rams and wethers suffer terribly and die within forty-eight hours, at most, on account of the bursting of the bladder.

While these roots have proven so fatal to rams and wethers the writer has fed mangels and sugar beets extensively during many seasons to breeding ewes and has never experienced any trouble therefrom. This is probably due to the fact that in rams and wethers the urinary canal is no more than about one-sixteenth inch in diameter, and the small stones forming in the bladder cannot pass through the canal. The ewes, however, have a much larger urinary canal, permitting the escape of the stones.

FLUSHING THE EWES.

A breeding ewe, if expected to uphold her vitality and vigor, needs a vacation once a year. She may have been a good mother, a heavy milker, and have raised one, two, or perhaps even three lambs. Although she has had good care and pasture she will naturally be run down somewhat in condition, because the greatest portion of the feed she has consumed has been utilized for the production of milk. She therefore needs a rest before she is bred again, and the time for her vacation will be between the weaning and breeding periods. During this time the breeding ewe ought to be what is commonly termed "flushed." Flushing means bringing the ewe from a thin condition into a good, strong, vigorous condition in a short time. When this is done the breeding ewe will be in the proper condition to assume her duty again when the breeding time arrives.

Flushing is highly recommended, for it has several advantages. How can a ewe which has been suckling her lamb all summer be brought into proper shape to take up her new burden at breeding time unless her lamb is weaned and she is flushed before she is bred? If bred in a thin, rundown condition she must resume work again immediately and will probably be brought into winter quarters thin and weak. In such condition she will be subject to many more diseases. She will be so delicate that any little cold which may attack her in this condition is liable to cause her death, while another ewe in good condition will resist the attack.

Another benefit that may be of interest, which is derived from the practice of flushing ewes, is the fact that to a certain extent the flockmaster following this practice has control over the percentage of lambs dropped by his ewes the following lambing time. It has been found that whenever ewes and rams are mated that are both in a strong, vigorous condition and full of vim more twins and triplets may be expected. These results can, however, only be obtained when both sire and dam are in good condition. If the ram is in good condition and the ewe is thin, or if the reverse is the case, then these results cannot be accomplished. Both ram and ewe must be vigorous and strong.

Another point in favor of having the ewes flushed before breeding is the fact that when properly flushed the flock of ewes will all breed within a shorter time, thus shortening up the lambing period. This will save the shepherd much loss of sleep.

The writer does not know of any feed that will flush ewes better and more cheaply than rape. This plant, when fully matured, will not lead to bloat in sheep. When the lower leaves on the stem begin to turn yellow, as well as the tips of the upper leaves, the rape is ripe and matured, and it may now be fed with safety. The rape seems to stimulate the inner organs of the sheep, making the ewes vigorous and strong and causing them to regain flesh. If, however, no rape has been grown for this purpose the next best feed is grain, which is of course more expensive. Oats have proved satisfactory, and cabbage may also be recommended.

CULLING THE EWE FLOCK.

Before breeding is to begin in the fall, the flock ought to be culled. All ewes that have not proved to be good producers and do not furnish enough milk to raise at least one good lamb should be the first to be culled out. All other ewes that have broken mouths, or whose udders or teats have accidentally become spoiled, should be sold to the butcher while still in a fleshy condition. At this time the shepherd must judge as to which ewes ought to be disposed of and which ought to be retained. He knows every individual and knows their records of production perhaps better than the owner of the flock himself, who may make it a point to inspect the flock but once in a while. Such men make mistakes very easily as they generally select the best looking ewes to be retained and dispose of the thin looking ones, not knowing that the fat ones did not give much milk, and consequently are in fine trim at this time. Let the shepherd, who knows each ewe and knows what she has done, do the culling, rather than someone else who is not so familiar with the flock.

CULLING THE LAMB FLOCK.

Later in the fall the lamb flock should also be culled. For the further improvement of the flock all the best ewe lambs should be reserved each

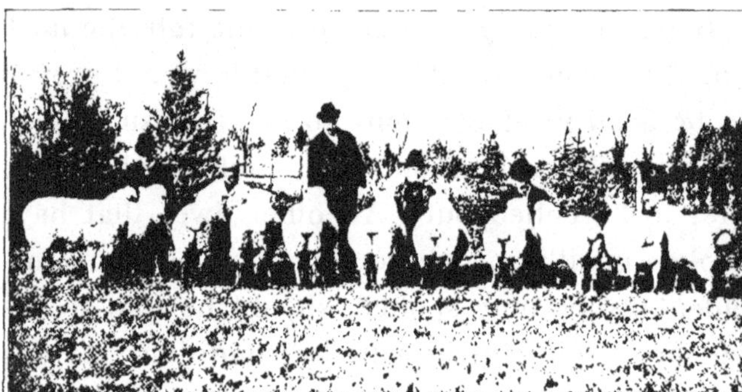

PLATE 41. A group of yearling wethers fitted at the University of Wisconsin for classroom demonrtration, 1898.

year, to take the place of the ewes that are culled out and sold. We often hear of men who sell their best ewe lambs and keep the inferior ones, simply because the butcher pays a cent or so more per pound for those of the more desirable class. This is poor policy, and the owner is the loser in the end. All other spare lambs may be sold when the market is good and the prices high.

CARE AT BREEDING TIME.

The proper time to breed in the fall depends entirely upon the judgment of the flockowner. If he has warm quarters for early-born lambs, ewes may be bred early; if such quarters cannot be provided, it is better not to have the lambs come so soon. Another factor which determines the time of breeding is whether lambs are to be sold for early or for late market. The breeder must suit himself, and should act according to existing conditions.

Before the ram is allowed to come to the ewes they should be nicely tagged. This means clipping all surplus wool off from the end of the tail, which materially aids the ram in mating with the ewes and saves his vitality. It also insures less barren ewes in the flock. The general appearance of a flock of ewes is also greatly improved if they are properly tagged.

NECESSITY OF SALT.

It has been stated elsewhere that sheep should have access to salt at all times of the year, for salt is an absolute necessity for them and when they are deprived of it great loss sometimes results. Salt furnishes chlorine for the digestive juices of the stomach and is also required for the proper functioning of many of the body organs. If salt is not supplied the digestion of the sheep will be impaired and serious consequences will follow. Sheep crave salt, and when it is given to them only once in a while they will usually eat too much at one time. They will then drink excessive amounts of water, which will upset the digestive organs and often cause severe scouring. If salt is supplied in abundance at all times, at no time will the sheep consume an excessive amount. Therefore, if all is to go well in the flock, one must not fail to provide salt every day of the year.

KEEP DOWN BURDOCKS AND SANDBURS.

Burdocks and sandburs are bitter enemies to the watchful flockmaster. When he notices that some of the sheep have collected any of these mean burs, he becomes alarmed, knowing that the appearance of his flock is much injured. But this is not all. He also realizes that the value of the wool is lessened when it comes to selling it, since buyers greatly object to wool in such a condition. Again, suppose the shepherd wants to show some of his sheep at the county fair. Can he do it when their fleeces are matted together with these burs? He may show them but they will not win any prizes, as the fleeces of prize winners must be in good, clean condition. The judge will not injure his hands on such sheep by handling them, instead he will pass them by. The writer has seen such sheep at county fairs, but he did not prick his fingers by handling them. If a shepherd wants to trim his sheep a little, how can he do it if these burs are present in the fleece? It may be done by spending a great deal of time picking them out, but this is a very slow and unpleasant job, and after much picking the shepherd cannot even then get the fleece into proper shape, to say nothing about spoiling his sheep shears.

When the first sheep is noticed carrying some of these pests a thorough search should be made over the field in which the sheep are pasturing, and wherever these miserable weeds are found they should be cut down and burned, and should then be fought to a finish until they are all destroyed. The writer has never believed in Sunday work, except performing the necessary chores, as the day belongs to God and in the writer's opinion no man has ever gained much by doing work on Sunday that should be done on Saturday or Monday. However, if on walking through the sheep pasture on Sunday he should see a clump of burdocks, he would immediately take out his jack-knife and destroy them, because he despises them so much. Of course, if there were many of them he would not meddle with them on Sunday, but would go after them on Monday morning before breakfast.

DANGERS OF DEAD FURROWS.

The writer wishes to call the attention of the beginner in the sheep business to the fact that when the sheep are turned out on pasture it is a wise

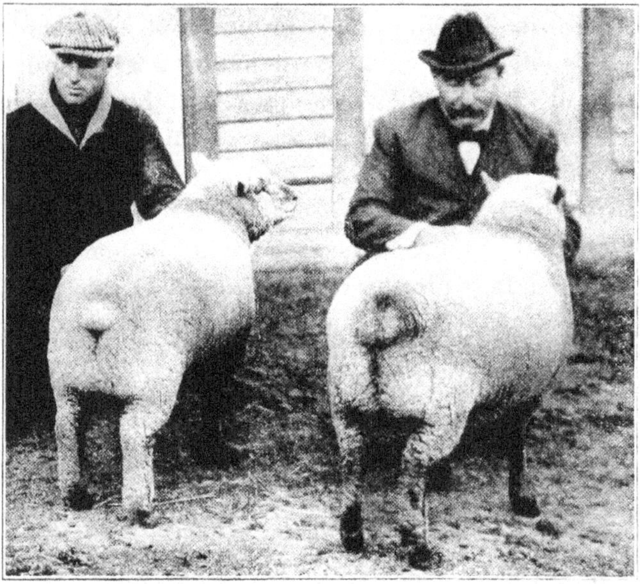

PLATE 45. Pure-bred Southdown yearling wethers. The one at the left won first prize and championship and reserve grand championship. The one at the right won third prize. Shown by the University of Wisconsin at the International, 1916.

plan to look over the land to see if there are any traps for them, that is, whether there are any shallow depressions, such as dead furrows, in the field where the flock pastures. In such depressions sheep like to lie down, especially over night.

These little hollows are exceedingly dangerous, especially if they are not much wider than the sheep, because sheep when lying down will sometimes roll over on their backs and on account of the small space will find it impossible to turn back again. The ground on both sides is higher, thus affording the sheep no chance of getting up again, and after lying in this position for two or three hours it will die. Dead furrows in fields are perhaps the most dangerous places for sheep to be trapped this way.

It is discouraging to find a plump, broad-backed ewe or lamb lying dead in one of these ditches or dead furrows, with its four legs standing straight up in the air. One will never find a thin, narrow-backed sheep lying on its back, but in every instance it is one of the very best in the flock. It is taken for granted that older flockmasters need not be warned to be cautious in this respect, for they have probably long ago learned through experience the danger of such dead furrows and ditches. It is an old saying that experience is the best teacher. True enough, but the lesson learned through self-experience is very often the most expensive one. How can the beginner with sheep be expected to know all about small details if he has not been warned by some one who has gone through the mill and has paid for his grinding?

If men who have had long years of experience and who take all the necessary precautions, sometimes stumble, how many more mistakes must the beginner make?

NUMBER OF SHEEP TO THE ACRE.

The question is often asked as to how many sheep can be pastured on an acre. This is difficult to answer since some acres produce three times as much feed as others. It is generally admitted that where one cow can be successfully pastured throughout a season, from five to eight sheep can be pastured. Since the larger breeds require more feed, from five to six head could be pastured on this area, while of the smaller ones as many as eight could find sufficient feed. However, no positive statement can be made in this regard.

CHAPTER VIII.

FEEDING SHEEP FOR MARKET.

Feeding sheep for market has proved very profitable to the men who have followed it extensively for a number of years. Some men, however, when newly starting in the business, struck one or two seasons that were not profitable, and consequently gave up this work in disgust, declaring it a failure. Many men, when they see others making money in any line of business, will jump into the same work, with the wrong idea that they are as well qualified for the undertaking and are just as capable of solving the problems as those who have learned the business through years of experience. Those who know the ups and downs through practice have reached the point where they can obtain a handsome profit almost any season by sheep feeding. Some years there is a large margin, and others a smaller one, but, on the average, men feeding sheep for market have made considerable money, and some have acquired great wealth from this source. However, the profit that can be derived from the undertaking depends largely upon the purchase price of the sheep, the prices of feed, and last but not least, the kind of market. If feeders are very high-priced in the fall one cannot expect a large margin over the purchase price, feed, and labor, unless high prices for finished mutton are realized.

In the Eastern and Middle States not as many sheep and lambs are annually fed as in the Western States. Michigan perhaps leads in the East, while Colorado is foremost in the West. However, smaller numbers of them are fed for market in nearly every state. Since the writer cannot discuss the large feeding operations in the West from personal experience, he will confine his discussion of the subject to the home industry where sheep are fed for market on a smaller scale. In many sections of the country a considerable number of men feed one or two carloads each winter. Others may just be starting in, and it is to these that the writer wishes to speak in particular.

AGE OF SHEEP TO BE FED.

It is generally admitted among feeders that lambs bring more profit when put in the feed lot than older sheep, for the simple reason that it requires less pounds of feed to produce a pound of gain in lambs than in yearlings or still older sheep. The lamb in the feed lot is not only putting on flesh, but is at the same time growing in size, while the older sheep though spreading and developing more in width of body and also putting on flesh, is actually not growing in size any more after it reaches the age of two years. Wherever practicable, it will pay the feeder to secure lambs for feeding, unless, of course, he can get yearlings or two-year-olds at a very low cost, which will enable him to realize a good profit from his investment. Fat lambs are in greater demand on the market than older sheep, and are therefore generally higher in price.

SELECTION OF FEEDERS.

In selecting feeders one ought to be very careful to get sound, healthy sheep and not buy a lot that is probably infested with internal parasites, as stomach or tape worms, or with scab or foot rot. If the feeder is not watchful he will cut his profit down right at the beginning by losing some of the sheep which were unsound when bought. He should therefore examine their eyes and skin, as has been explained in a previous chapter of this work, in order to make sure that they do not have parasites. Many feeders prefer range sheep to natives, since range sheep are generally free from internal parasites. If they are only infested with ticks or lice they may easily be freed from these pests by dipping them, but it will be a more difficult task to cure them of skin diseases or internal parasites. It is also unprofitable to meddle with sheep that have old, broken mouths and are therefore unable to chew their feed properly and hence must have all the grain ground for them. It has further been learned that sheep or lambs that are in pretty fair condition when they are placed in the feed lot make better gains than those that are in too thin a condition at the time. In a trial at the Wisconsin Station, lambs accustomed to grain from the time of birth were able to make a weekly gain of 3.8 pounds per head for a period of twelve weeks feeding. Other lambs, not receiving any grain until they were put in the feed lot in the fall, with the most judicious care and feeding only gained 2.5 pounds per head per week for the same length of time. The first lot made a net profit of $1.40 per head, while the others made only $.80 per head.

In all cases a class of sheep should be obtained that have good, wide body frames, that are broad and low-down to the ground, and that have broad heads. Pay no attention to the long-legged, narrow-bodied, long-necked, and slim-faced class, as they require more feed to produce a pound of gain in weight than the right class will, and are therefore less profitable to feed. Of course, it is well understood that the feeder cannot always get exactly what he is striving to secure, but he should not be satisfied to obtain a class that will not give him the largest net returns from the feeding operation.

When purchased by a carload or more, some of the sheep or lambs will be larger than the others. The larger ones generally take advantage of the smaller ones at the feed trough and push them back, and in this way get more than their share of the feed. To give them all an equal chance a good plan is to group them in two or more lots, each size by itself. They usually do much better in smaller lots than when too many are bunched together.

THE PRINCIPLES OF FEEDING.

Some feeders do not obtain as good results as others, simply because they have not yet learned the few underlying principles which, when carefully observed, lead to success.

1. *Gentleness and patience.*—A sheep is frightened very easily. Therefore, the feeder in charge must not be one of the coarse, rough men who will make his way into the feed lot by kicking and pounding the sheep that get in his way. Gentle treatment counts for a great deal in this line of work, since sheep make more and cheaper gains when treated kindly. Many a time the writer has had his cap or hat pulled off from his head when

stooping down to clean out feed troughs, but nevertheless the lambs were not abused for so doing. On the contrary the feeder rather enjoys this playfulness, because he feels that the lambs have full confidence in him and fear no harm.

The good feeder should also be patient. It often happens that an inquisitive lamb will stand with its front feet in the trough and perhaps soil it somewhat, just after it has been cleaned out nicely before feeding. The patient feeder in this case will not run after the lamb and try to make it understand that this act was wrong. He will reclean the trough and say nothing. Sheep will always well repay the kind treatment that is shown them. The man who rushes into the feed lot without warning the sheep of his approach by speaking to them, so that they will not become frightened and run for doors and windows to get away from him as far as possible, is and will always be a poor feeder until he begins to change his ways. Any man who does not care for sheep should never be allowed to feed them, as he will certainly not make good.

2. *Cleanliness.*—At all times it is necessary to practice cleanliness. Sheep dc not require as much feed as other classes of live stock, but this comparatively small amount must by all means be clean, for sheep are more particular as to what

they eat than most farm animals. It will never do to try to make them eat grain that has been scratched over by the chickens many times and is soiled. Nor can they under ordinary circumstances be forced to eat some of the commercial feeds, or hay that has a bad odor. The feed troughs must, furthermore, be thoroughly cleaned out before each meal and must always be kept in a sweet condition. Have you ever noticed that wherever there are a few droppings of a sheep in the feed trough sheep will eat all the clean grain around this place, but will not touch the soiled grain that is on or near it? It will certainly pay any feeder to practice cleanliness, as the sheep itself is a clean animal.

3. *Punctuality.*—By punctuality we mean in this case that a certain time be scheduled for feeding each day, and for each meal in particular. This time should be fixed definitely right at the start. Brother feeder, have you ever stopped to realize the importance of punctuality in sheep feeding? Have you ever considered how much better and cheaper gains can be made in feeding when the time set for each meal is strictly adhered to?

Visit a good feeder, get into deep conversation with him on some important subject, and try to make him forget the time for feeding his sheep. You will notice him pulling out his watch every

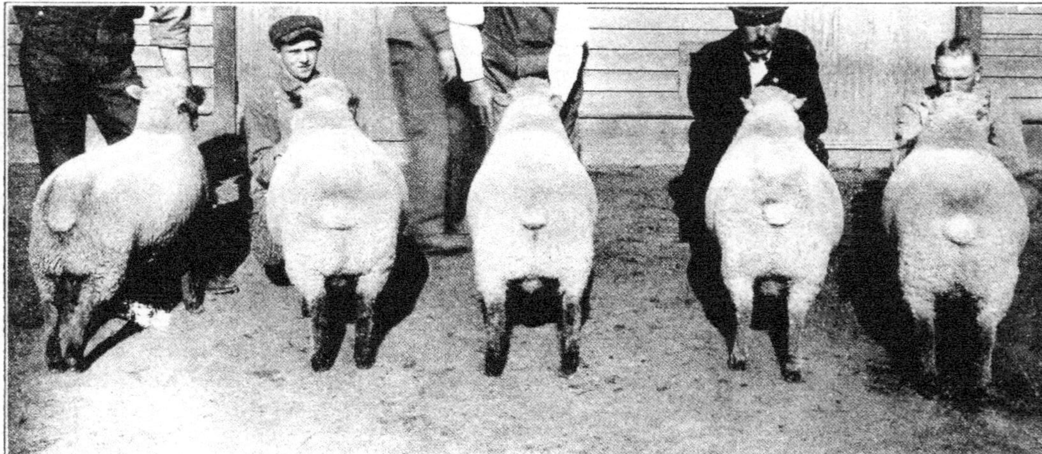

PLATE 46. Pen of five grade yearling wethers. Winners of first prize in the open and also in the college class Shown by the University of Wisconsin at the International, 1917

little while to see whether the time for feeding has come, and when the hour has arrived he will undoubtedly ask to be excused so that he may do his feeding. He is aware of the fact that his sheep are accustomed to getting their meals at a certain fixed time, and that when the feeder fails to be on hand the sheep begin to bleat and worry and wonder what could have happened to their feeder. The longer the delay after the regular feeding hour, the more flesh they worry off, instead of putting on. Remember that your profit will depend a good deal on the value and importance you place upon punctuality in feeding.

Another point of great value is that the feeding should be done as quickly as possible. Grain, the feed which is eaten up the most rapidly, is generally fed first. Roughage is fed last of all, in order to give the sheep ample time to pick it over and allow the feeder to get through so that he can perform other urgent work. It would certainly not be very wise to give them their grain ration, which is eaten up in a short time, and in the meantime go away and forget all about giving them their next ration. Such action would be absolutely unprofitable. Feed them their grain, if so planned, and when this is cleaned up, the next ration, and so on until all is given them that is to be fed at one meal. After they have eaten their full ration allow them to lie down and rest undisturbed until the next meal time. This will give them plenty of time to chew their cud and properly digest their meal. It has been found at the Wisconsin Station that feeding fattening lambs only twice a day is sufficient, and is even more conducive to rapid growth than feeding three times daily. As sheep are mostly fattened in the winter time when the days are short it is well to begin feeding about six o'clock A. M. and again at four o'clock P. M., making it entirely unnecessary to feed them at noon.

4. *Judgment.*—The person who does the sheep feeding should be one who likes sheep. There is no sense whatever in trying to have a man feed sheep who dislikes them or who possesses no judgment. The feeder's ability and judgment are shown in every case of success or failure. The careful feeder watches all the members in the lot of sheep closely, studies their appetites, and feeds them just enough so as to prevent overfeeding at any one meal. He begins lightly and gradually increases their feed, for if they are overfed at one meal they will often scour and may then lose as much in live weight in three days as can be restored in the following two weeks. Scouring will also make the wool filthy, thus greatly injuring the appearance of the sheep and reducing the price of the wool.

The same person should always do the feeding. If by accident an unfamiliar person who is not acquainted with the capacity of the sheep in his charge and the proper allowance to be given them is allowed to do the feeding at any time he is apt to upset the whole lot. One feeder also may be able to feed economically, while another may be wasteful. For example, sheep make their best gains in fairly cold weather when the temperature is nearly down to zero. If they are then on full feed they may be pushed along steadily. But if now all at once warm weather sets in the well-posted feeder will cut down on the grain ration, because he knows that sheep, especially lambs, cannot stand as much grain in warm weather as in cold weather. On the other hand, the feeder who is ignorant of this fact will feed the same amount with the result that he gets them off feed, and it is a difficult matter to have them regain their appetite when once it is lost. Not much can be accomplished when the same person does not do the feeding each day, as the one is liable to spoil what the other has accomplished. In all cases feeding grain must be begun lightly in order to avoid overfilling and scouring.

LITTLE EXERCISE FOR FATTENING SHEEP.

It has already been stated that too much exercise cannot be given to pregnant ewes. Sheep when being fattened for market do not, however, need much exercise. They may be given a little exercise now and then, but in general they gain faster if not allowed to run about at all, but if kept closely confined to their quarters.

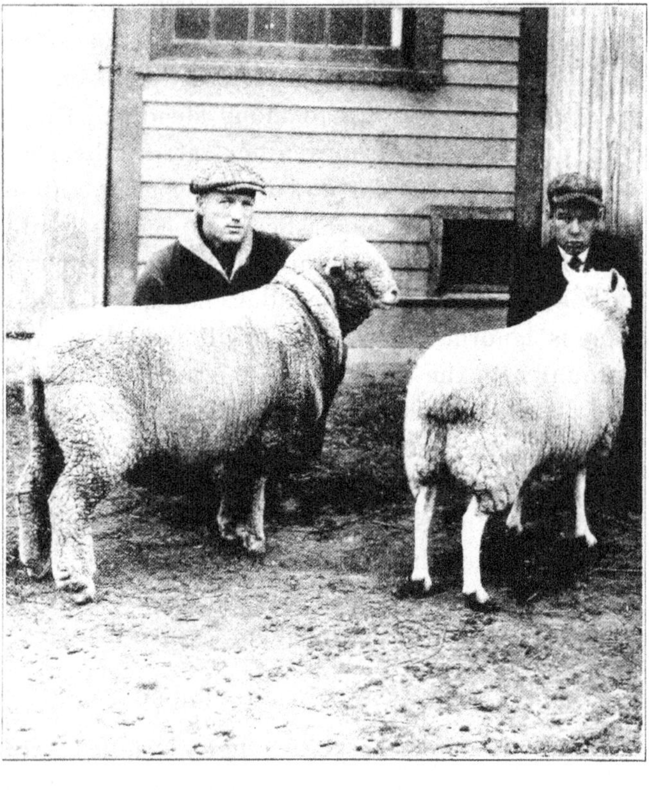

PLATE 47. First prize and champion Cheviot yearling wether at the right; first prize and champion yearling Rambouillet wether at the left, at the International, 1916. Shown by the University of Wisconsin.

HAND-FEEDING OR SELF-FEEDERS.

Where a large number of sheep or lambs are fed at any one place and good feeders of sheep are scarce it is perhaps feasible to employ self-feeders, for by the use of self-feeders a great deal of hand labor is saved. Where smaller lots are being fed, however, hand-feeding can be much more highly recommended, since sheep are greedy, and when they have free access to the grain they often eat too much of it. In many instances a large number of lambs have been lost on account of overloaded stomachs caused by eating too much grain.

The writer at one time visited a large feeding plant and counted as many as eleven dead lambs one morning. When the man in charge was questioned as to the cause of death, his reply was that the self-feeders had killed them by allowing them to eat too much grain. The writer was informed that out of the two thousand lambs in the feed lot some were lost every day through the use of self-feeders. The danger of eating too much grain is prevented when hand-feeding is practiced. Where large numbers are fed, and labor is high, however, the large operator cannot be blamed for using self-feeders.

SHELTER.

Whenever possible, shelter should be provided for the fattening sheep. Yet at many western feeding yards no shelter whatever is given the sheep. But when sheep are not sheltered their fleeces at times become soaking wet from rains or snows, and the result is lung trouble and pneumonia. They do not, however, need a warm or very costly place. All that is necessary is a simple roof over them to keep them dry. Do not allow feeding sheep or any others to wade or sleep in a yard where the mud is perhaps knee deep. Any kind of sheep like to have it dry underneath them, and comfortable dry quarters help them materially to put on flesh.

GRAIN FOR FATTENING.

Many large feeding operators have used wheat screenings chiefly as the grain ration. The writer is unable to say anything relative to the feeding value of wheat screenings, as they have never been used at this Station for the reason that they contain large amounts of weed seeds, which will get into the manure in spite of the greatest care and be brought into the fields, there causing havoc. The best and cheapest returns in different trials conducted at this Station have been obtained by feeding shelled corn, provided corn is available at a normal price. Dried beet pulp also has given very satisfactory results, and stands almost equal to corn in feeding value for sheep, besides being much cheaper. Oats, when used as the sole grain, have never given much profit in fattening sheep or lambs. In every instance the cost price of the different grains must be considered as well as their actual feeding value.

As already stated, nice corn stands about first in rank in fattening sheep. Sheep will soon get tired of pure corn feeding, however, and the best feeders do not therefore find it an easy matter to feed it alone for any great length of time, and have the sheep progress as they should. For this reason it is advisable to mix a little oats and bran with the corn, in order to have a more balanced ration. Where the grain for fattening sheep is grown on the farm no better ration can be recommended than a mixture of four parts of shelled corn, one part of oats, and one part of bran. Toward the last three or four weeks before marketing, a little oilmeal may be added to finish them off. Barley is likewise of great value for this purpose.

Throughout the Western range district, where corn is not raised in large quantities, barley is extensively used for fattening sheep and lambs. Trials conducted at the Montana and South Dakota Experiment Stations show that when fed as the only grain allowance to fattening range lambs whole barley was only slightly less valuable than corn.

Wheat should not be fed to fattening sheep except when off grade or extremely low in price, as it tends to produce growth rather than fat. Trials at the South Dakota Station show that durum or macaroni wheat has about the same value as bread wheat.

Like wheat, oats tend to produce growth, and therefore it is not best to use them as the sole grain for fattening. As already stated a little oats will help to balance up corn or barley.

Owing to the greatly increased production of emmer, or speltz, in the Western States, this grain has gained some importance as a feed for fattening sheep and lambs. Trials at the South Dakota Station showed that with prairie or brome hay emmer was much less valuable than corn. In a trial at the Colorado Station, however, emmer made unusually economical gains when fed with good alfalfa hay.

Feeds which are rich in crude protein, such as linseed meal, cotton-seed meal, field peas, and soybeans, may sometimes be profitably mixed with corn or other grains for fattening lambs or sheep. Care must be used in feeding these heavy rich feeds.

ROUGHAGES FOR FATTENING.

The legume hays furnish the best roughages for fattening sheep. In the East flockowners may raise clover or alfalfa, those in the South cowpeas and perhaps alfalfa, and those in the West alfalfa. In Colorado, where in 1907 two million lambs and sheep were fed, the standard ration is alfalfa hay and corn, these feeds forming about ninety-five per cent of all the feed used.

Good pea straw, and also bean straw, are relished by sheep. Of recent years a few sheep have been successfully fattened on pea-cannery refuse, together with grain. In some sections of the West, especially in the San Luis Valley, Colorado, many lambs and sheep are grazed on field peas. The sheep are turned on the peas as soon as they mature, and without other feed are fattened in from 70 to 120 days.

As before stated, timothy or marsh hay should never be offered to sheep if other roughage can be secured. Good, bright, fine oat straw is preferable to either of these roughages.

SUCCULENT FEEDS.

Succulent feeds, such as roots and corn silage, are valuable in feeding sheep for market. In the writer's experience roots not only keep the digestive organs of sheep in good condition but also make considerable gain and increase the yolk in the wool to quite an extent. Not much additional gain can be expected from feeding corn silage to lambs,

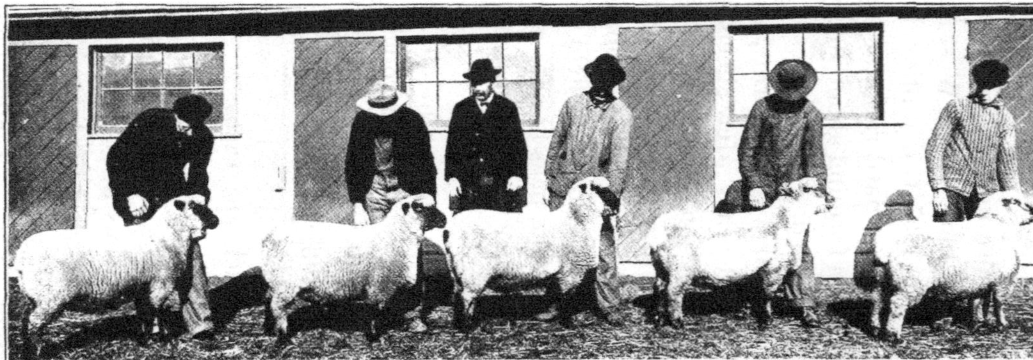

PLATE 48. Pen of grade Shropshire yearling wethers which won first prize at the International, 1909, shown by the University of Wisconsin.

but this feed also is valuable in keeping the digestive organs in good condition.

Near beet sugar factories wet beet pulp has proved to be satisfactory for fattening lambs when fed with such feeds as alfalfa hay and corn.

RAPE FEEDING PREVIOUS TO FATTENING.

From trials carried on at this Station it has been found that very cheap gains have been made by feeding rape previous to placing the sheep in the feed lot. If a piece of rape is sown not later than July 1 it will come in handy to turn the sheep onto before they are placed in the feed lot. In an experiment conducted at this Station lambs pastured on rape, but fed no grain, made as large gains as others on good grass pasture and fed one pound of grain daily but no rape. In other words one pound of grain was saved by each lamb daily, and the lambs on rape made just as much gain as the other lambs that received one pound of grain. It was further learned when finishing both lots off on dry feed that the lambs which had received rape previously did considerably better than the other lot not receiving rape before being put into the feed lot. The writer must say that he has always placed great faith in rape as a cheap and valuable feed for sheep.

BEST TIME TO MARKET

Lambs are generally fed from sixty to ninety days before marketing, depending upon the condition they are in when put into the feed lot. The prices on the market must also be taken into consideration. If lambs are to be marketed early in the season the feeding should be commenced early, so that they may be ready just about the time when the rush to market in the fall is over. There are times when there is a notable scarcity on the market, one of which is between the marketing of the grass-fed and the winter-fed lot, from about December 10 to January 10. At this time lambs usually sell for high prices, since the grass lambs have all come to market and most of those put in the feed lot are not ready for market. By having the lambs ready for market at this time strong competition may be avoided. If a late market is decided upon the feeding may be started late, so as to get the lambs on the market when most feeding yards are exhausted, namely in the latter part of March and April. Although a high-priced market cannot be guaranteed for these times every year, still, on the average, comparatively high prices are paid at this period of the year. Always try to bring your stuff to market when the other fellow is not there, so as to avoid competition.

Feeders often make a mistake in marketing their lambs before they are fat. Sheep or lambs that are not in a fat condition when brought to the market, or so-called "half-fed" stuff, are often sold at a sacrifice. Butchers are willing to pay high prices for prime animals, but are just as unwilling to pay much for stuff only half fat. This class of sheep suffers from depression in price at nearly all times of the year.

Large, heavy ewes are invariably considered a drug on the market, while lambs weighing from eighty to ninety pounds and in prime condition are readily sold at good prices. The eighty-five pound lamb is in greater demand on the market than the one hundred pound lamb. Packers claim that the one hundred pound lamb is not as profitable to them as what is termed the "handy weight" lamb.

In a lot of fattening lambs some will always thrive better and put on flesh more rapidly than others. Therefore, when some of them have been properly fattened and prices are right, these should be selected and shipped and the thinner ones should be retained and fed until they also have become fat.

Before marketing lambs clip all loose locks of wool off from their sides and necks, caused by rubbing against each other on the feed troughs or crowding each other at meal time. Also tag them nicely around the tail. When this is done at least ten per cent will be added to their selling price. Expert buyers do not judge by looks alone, and they thoroughly handle the sheep before bidding on them. Yet the clean, broad, and square appearance of a lamb at its rear adds greatly to the selling price. Never forget that a good looking bunch of lambs or sheep on the market will always attract the eye of the buyer.

HOW TO FEED BEFORE SHIPPING.

It is a very foolish practice to fill lambs up on feed to their utmost capacity before loading them for market. Some feeders believe that they will gain by stuffing the lambs before loading, but this is not the case. When they are filled up in such manner, many will begin to scour before reaching the market, and will have a very disagreeable and filthy appearance when they arrive. Such lambs will also shrink more in weight than those fed only their regular ration, or even less. Even with proper feeding before loading the shaking they get in transit in freight cars, and the puffing and the noise of the engine,—quite a change of conditions from the quiet home from whence they have come, —is sufficient to upset their stomachs, and if they are overloaded with feed beforehand matters are much worse. They will look cleaner, brighter, and fresher when coming out of the car if fed only on dry feed before being loaded, and not even a full meal at that. When fed lightly they will drink water upon their arrival at the stock yards and will look just about as good as they did at home, and the shrinkage will be comparatively small.

Another mistake that is very often made is crowding too many lambs into one car. What is the result? First, it is hard on the animals, and second, it means another loss to the shipper. When there is not sufficient standing room in the car and the lambs are packed together like sardines, the larger and stronger lambs will free themselves by jumping on top of the others, but what becomes of those underneath? They will patiently bear the load as long as possible. Their strength, however, gives away before they reach their destination, and they sink to the floor and suffocate. More than once the writer has seen stock cars opened at stock yards in which from three to seven lambs were found dead, due to overcrowding in the car. Is there any profit in this? Is it not cruel to subject poor, innocent lambs to such a terrible death? No intelligent feeder or shipper will allow himself to be guilty of such actions.

WINTER LAMBS.

Where the chief object is to raise lambs for market, there is in the writer's opinion no way to make

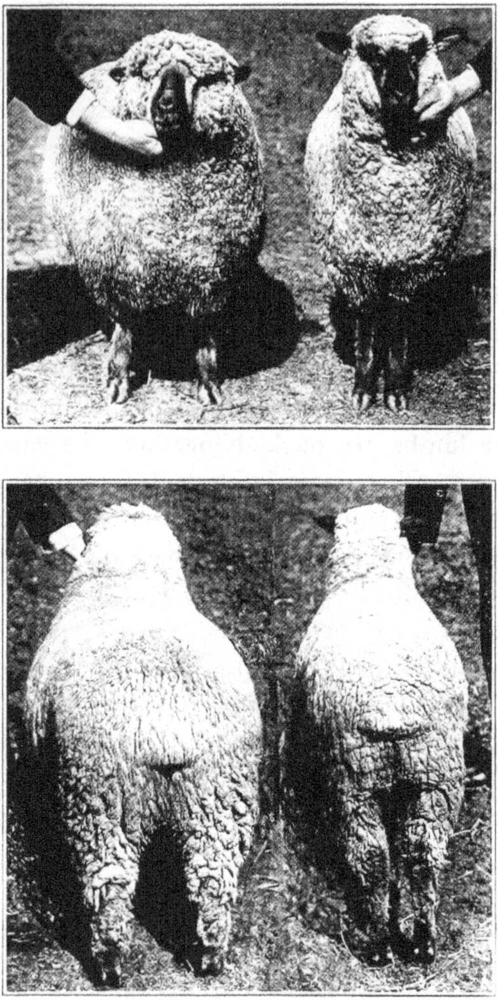

PLATE 13. Two grade Shropshire wether lambs showing the result of the use of a good and an inferior sire.

money faster than by raising winter, or so-called "hot-house" lambs. The winter lamb is born in the fall in the months of October and November, while lambs are usually born in the spring. With proper care these lambs can be gotten ready for market during the winter, from Christmas to Easter, at a time when young, juicy lamb is a scarcity, and such meat will bring high prices in the markets of the large cities.

In order to raise winter lambs we must have ewes that can be bred from about the middle of March till the first of July. Nearly all breeds of sheep take the ram in the fall and lamb in the spring, and it is rarely possible to make them reverse the order of nature.

Various methods have been advocated to get any breed of ewes to breed in the spring and summer. Some claimed that when ewes were taken in the spring or summer and kept in a cold place, such as an ice-house, for about a week they would breed. Another method advocated was, after feeding the ewes in the morning, to drive them all day long on a shady road. When this had been repeated each day for a week it was claimed the ewes would surely breed. Still another method was to feed the ewes very highly, giving them all they would eat of the richest grain, besides hay or other feeds. At the end of a week they were to be fed on a very scant ration, such as oat straw, with little or nothing else. After these two weeks, one of high living and the other of almost starvation, they were again fed an abundance of the richest feeds

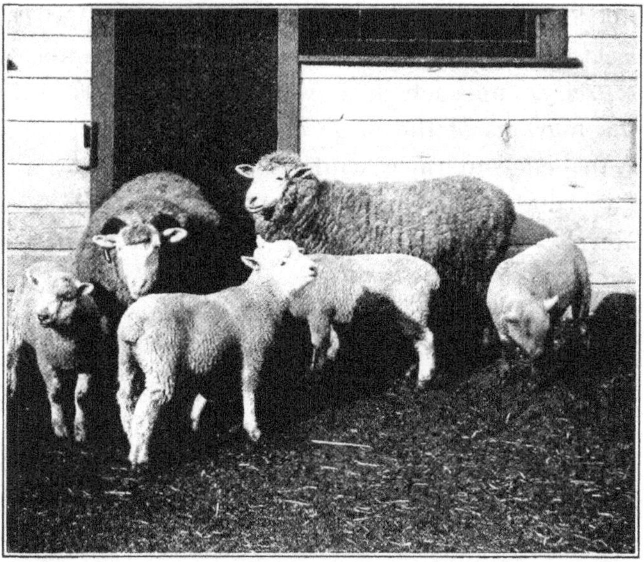

PLATE 50. Two grade Dorset ewes with their four winter lambs at the University of Wisconsin.

and were supposed to breed immediately. All of these artificial methods have been tried by the writer, but none of them proved to be at all successful, which emphasizes the difficulty of working against nature. However, the ewes of one breed of sheep, the Dorset Horn, naturally breed in the spring or early summer. This breed of sheep is therefore best adapted to the raising of winter lambs.

There is another breed of sheep, the Tunis, which it is claimed will breed in the spring like the Dorsets. However, the writer has had no experience with Tunis sheep and is therefore unable to make any statement concerning their merits in this respect.

While it has been said that Dorset ewes will breed in the spring and summer, it can also be said that some of them will breed twice in one year and thus drop two crops of lambs. At this Station some years ago a Dorset ram was crossed on grade Shropshire ewes, and the majority of the ewes from this first cross bred like pure-bred Dorsets in the early spring and again in the fall. In the accompanying illustration are shown two of these grade Dorset ewes and their lambs. The writer especially remembers one of these grade Dorset ewes which for two years in succession bred twice a year, dropped two lambs each time, and raised them all.

CARE OF DORSET EWES.

Dorset ewes before they are bred in the spring should be in good flesh and should be sheared as early as possible in the season. When the desired breeding time approaches a good, strong, vigorous ram should be turned with the flock and left with them all day and night. While this is perhaps contrary to what has been previously recommended, in this case it will help to get the ewes to breed more quickly, as the ram when left with the flock will tease the ewes.

If a Dorset flock of ewes is once established a ram of one of the other mutton breeds may be used. Of course, the ewe lambs could not then be kept for further winter lamb breeding, as they would tend to lose Dorset characteristics. Whatever breed the ram is, he should be a vigorous fellow and in thrifty condition.

In the summer months after the ewes have been bred they do not need any special care so long as they have plenty of good pasture. In the fall, however, when lambing time approaches and pastures usually get scant, the ewes should receive a little grain in order to insure a heavy milk flow. A warm place must be provided for these ewes to lamb in, since young lambs grow and thrive much better in general in a warm place than they do in a cold one. When a lamb lies down, curls up into a ball, and shivers from the cold it will not grow well. On the other hand, when it is nice and warm in their quarters and the lambs feel comfortable, get up and stretch themselves, play and jump, then they will thrive and do well.

The writer has learned during many years of experience with this breed of sheep, that compared with other breeds, the Dorsets are extremely heavy milkers. This may be due to the fact that a large flow of milk is necessary to feed the two or three lambs a Dorset ewe will usually have. As these ewes are such good mothers they need extra good feeding after lambing, especially if they are to have two crops of lambs in a year.

FEEDING THE WINTER LAMBS.

When the young lambs begin to eat, a good grain ration must be given them, such as is elsewhere mentioned in this book. Good alfalfa or second crop clover hay is also essential. Furthermore, if this line of work is to be carried on, roots, and especially cabbage, should be grown and stored so they may be fed to the mothers to increase their flow of milk, and to the lambs to make them grow as fast as possible. The writer has found that these young lambs relish cabbage, chopped up finely, more than any other feed he knows of. The lambs should receive their feed in a lamb creep, such as has been advocated for other lambs. When kept in good warm quarters, fed properly, and furnished by their mothers with an abundance of milk, the lambs can be made to gain five or six pounds per week. The writer has raised winter lambs which when fifty days old weighed fifty-five pounds, and others which weighed sixty-three pounds when sixty days old.

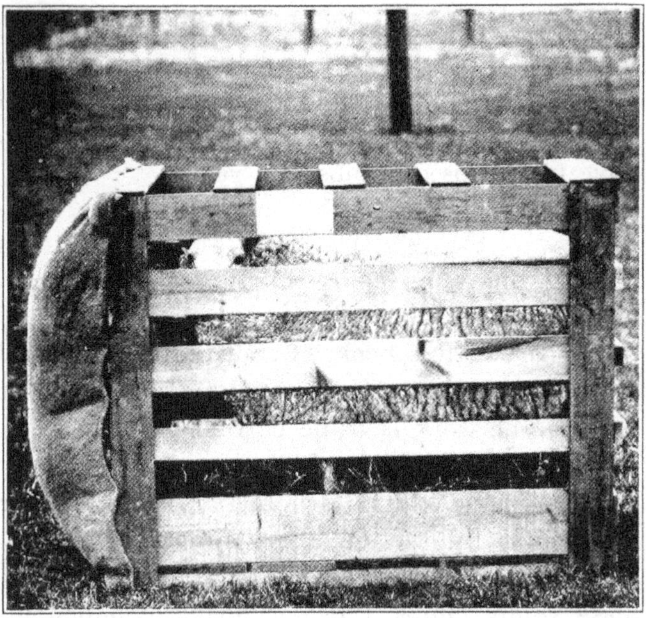

PLATE 51. A sheep properly crated for shipment. Note the bag at the front of the crate which contains the necessary feed for a long journey.

The desired weight for this class of lambs is from forty-five to sixty pounds, and they should sell for from fifteen to twenty cents per pound, live weight. Of course, the selling price will depend on the fatness and plumpness of the lamb, and the market.

In general such lambs will sell for a higher price in the Eastern markets than in the markets of the Middle-West. Quite a number of lambs raised at this Station have been sold on the Chicago market for from $10.00 to $13.00 per head at the age of sixty days or under. As Dorset ewes generally have twins, or even triplets, it can be seen that there is a great profit in this line of sheep husbandry. In the cases where ewes breed twice a year the profit is correspondingly larger. The writer wishes to emphasize the fact that where ewes raise two crops of lambs each year they must be well fed at all times, in order to uphold their vitality under the severe strain. Such ewes have been known to take the ram again when their suckling lambs were only three weeks old.

It has been found to be more profitable to dress the lambs before sending them to market than to ship them alive, for such young chaps shrink heavily in transit. Of course, when dressed at home. some such market as a hotel, a restaurant, or a meat market must be secured in advance and the dressed lambs shipped direct to that place. The lambs may either be fully dressed or rough dressed, that is, with the skin on the carcass, according to the requirements of the consumer.

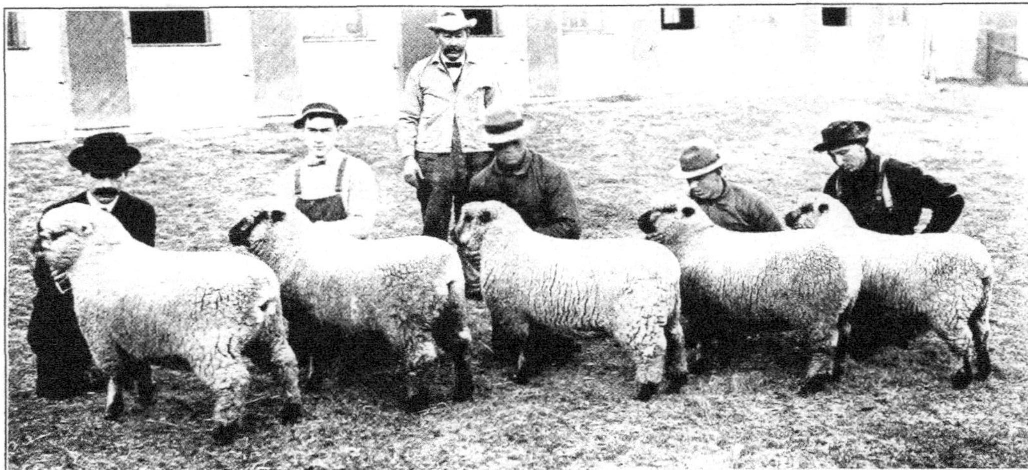

PLATE 52. First prize pen of grade Shropshire wether lambs at the International, 1908, shown by the University of Wisconsin.

CHAPTER IX.

FITTING SHEEP FOR THE SHOW RING.

While fitting and showing is pursued by comparatively few of the thousands of flockmasters, it may be helpful to outline briefly the principal details of the business for the benefit of the man who is thinking of taking up show fitting work. A number of shepherds have become famous and have gained a national reputation for themselves and their employers in the show ring. Many of these experts are well along in years now, and others must be trained in this work to take the place of the older men who will retire. It is to assist those who are beginners in fitting show sheep that the writer takes up the subject. But fitting show sheep can scarcely be learned from books to the point of becoming an expert, because no writer is able to put down all the small details which he follows and which have to be observed to be successful in the show ring. Therefore, after reading all one can find about fitting show sheep, the beginner should not expect to be as successful at the start as the man with many years of experience.

Some of the main obstacles for beginners may be avoided by learning from the experience of older show fitters. Not every one who started in this work can today look back with pride at his record. Many tried to fit and show once or twice, but today they are no longer in the race for they dropped out simply because they were not successful at the start. It seems as if only a small number of men naturally possess the necessary liking for sheep, the personal qualifications, and the unbounded persistency and self-sacrifice necessary to make a success of this work. For some men it is too tiresome a job, others have not enough patience to feed so carefully as is required to obtain the best results. Others find it too troublesome to be down on their knees a good deal of their time molding out a sheep with the shears to a perfect form.

"This work of fitting prize winners may be classed among the fine arts," said Prof. W. A. Henry at one time. This is indeed very true, and those who have practiced this line of work for years fully agree with this statement. Yet while there are many happy hours in the showman's life there are apt to be a great many more that are dark and gloomy. The sweet as well as the bitter medicine must be swallowed. No one can show more plainly whether he really is a man or not than when he meets with defeat in the show ring. Grumbling and disorderly conduct towards the judge or fellow exhibitors have never been of any benefit to the showman. If the exhibitor takes his lessons in the proper spirit he can gain knowledge

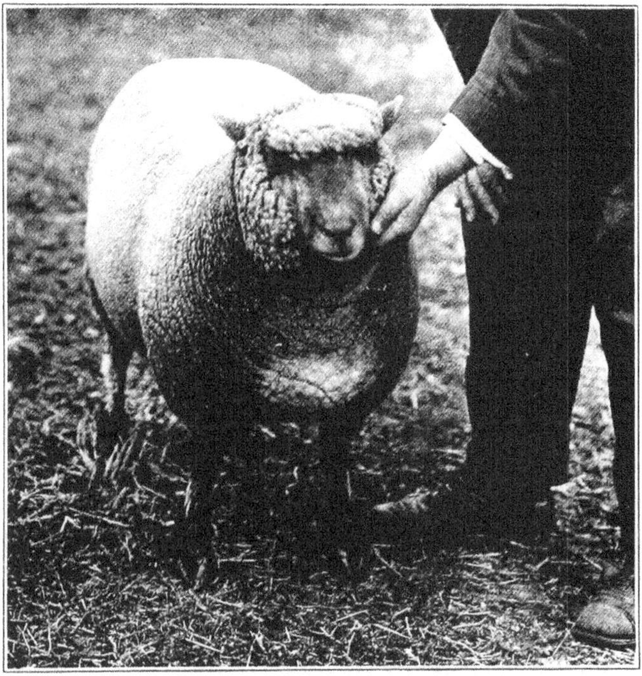

PLATE 53. Champion pure-bred Southdown yearling wether at the International, 1912. This wether was also the champion wether in the dressed carcass class. Shown by the University of Wisconsin.

faster in the show ring than anywhere else. Some exhibitors, however, always look at things in the wrong light and therefore do not learn the valuable lessons which may be learned in the show ring.

If beginners in fitting and showing sheep are earnest students in their undertaking, are reasonable, and are able to see things in the right light they can in time become just as successful as the older men who are securing the prizes at the present time.

It is not the writer's intention to discourage anyone from entering the field, by pointing out some of the dark clouds. On the contrary he wishes to urge all those who possess good judgment, who like the work, who are not afraid to put in extra hours, who have energy to do better work than others have done, and who are honest and faithful, to come forward and demonstrate their ability as loyal showmen. The beginner will not find the shepherds a mournful lot of fellows, but on the contrary, if he wishes to have a good time at shows and fairs, he should seek the company of the other shepherds after their working hours are over and listen to their stories and jokes. He will find them, as a rule, the happiest lot of fellows on the fair grounds.

CLASSES OF SHOW SHEEP

When we speak of fitting sheep for shows we have in mind two distinct classes, namely the breeding sheep that are to be shown in the breeding classes, and the fat sheep that are to be shown in the fat classes. There is quite a difference in the fitting and preparation of these two separate classes of sheep. The first class can be fitted in a much shorter time than the fat class, and the feeds for them are of a little different nature from those for the fat class.

SELECTION FOR THE BREEDING CLASS.

One of the chief factors in fitting sheep for breeding classes in the show ring is to be familiar with the up-to-date type and conformation of the breed or breeds to be fitted. No sheep, no matter how well it may be fitted, will be a winner if it does not possess the correct type, combined with the proper conformation and color. For instance a Shropshire ram that has stubs of horns should not win a prize, no matter how good an individual he may be in all other respects, for this is contrary to the standard of pure-bred Shropshires. Again a ram with only one testicle should not be fitted, for he will not win a prize if the judge is capable of discovering the lack. A sheep of any breed that is either undersized or too large for its particular breed also does not receive much consideration in the show ring. Neither does a sheep that has not the right color, or has a poor conformation, or has crooked legs, or is in too thin a condition, or on the contrary is too fat, get any recognition by the judge. Only the best ones in the flock should be selected. These should be true to type, of the right size and conformation, with the desirable kind of fleece and skin, with the four legs properly set under them, and with all the style and carriage possible. It never pays to fit sheep for the show ring that are not built right, or as is often said, born right, as the flesh and fitting alone will not bring the sheep to the front in the ring if they are lacking in these other respects. The competition is getting stronger year by year, and as a result greater care must be exercised each year in the selection and fitting of sheep for the show ring.

SHEARING SHEEP FOR THE BREEDING CLASSES.

It is common among exhibitors in the breeding classes to shear their sheep quite early in the spring, for in the show ring a long fleece is desirable on breeding sheep. For this reason, this class of sheep may be shorn as early as April 1, and a good length, growth, and staple of wool can then be had on the sheep at fair time. Some men shear even earlier than April 1, but the writer is of the opinion that sheep that are shorn too early have not as much brightness and lustre in their fleeces as those that are shorn at about the time stated. Moreover, in the hot summer weather sheep with too long fleeces do not do nearly as well as those that have shorter fleeces.

The old fashion of "stubble" shearing, which means taking only part of the wool off the sheep, should not be reverted to at all, because all experienced shepherds have found this to be a bad practice. Do not shear too early if a nice, thrifty-looking fleece is expected on a show sheep. The fine wool breeders are in the habit of shearing their Merinos in late fall and early winter. Although this breed of sheep does not show the effect of too early shearing quite as much as the middle and long wools do, nevertheless we occasionally meet some flocks of Merinos in the show ring whose fleeces are not in the proper "bloom," due to too early shearing.

PROPER TIME TO START FITTING.

The time to start fitting sheep intended for breeding classes depends upon the time they are to be shown. Two months to ten weeks brings sheep into good shape for these classes. However, the fitter must use his own judgment to know when they are in best condition to suit the judge. In other words, he must be a good judge of sheep himself. In the case of older sheep this may easily be decided by careful examination as to the condition the sheep are in. Lambs need fitting from the time of their birth.

FEED FOR SHOW LAMBS.

In order to keep lambs growing constantly they must always be given an abundance of feed. As soon as they are able to eat grain, they should receive it. They can also be given roots, good clover hay, and some cabbage or turnips. Rape should be sown early to feed to them at the time when pastures are getting short in the middle of summer. As long as the weather is cool the lambs do well on a grain ration consisting of bran, oats, a little cornmeal, and some oilmeal. However, when the weather begins to get hot too much corn must not be fed, for corn produces heat and makes lambs founder very easily. In the hot weather their ration should consist mostly of green feed. Some cracked field peas are very beneficial for fitting show sheep and lambs, as they produce a firm and solid flesh. In all cases lambs are much harder to fit than older sheep, as they are more tender and cannot withstand heavy feeding like older ones.

FEED FOR OLDER SHEEP.

The feed for older sheep is practically the same as for lambs, with the one exception that they can be fed more grain if it should be needed, for there is less danger of foundering them. In the hot weather it is a good plan to feed show sheep in a cool, airy barn during the day time and turn them out on good pasture during the night. This will give them the necessary exercise, which is absolutely indispensable in keeping them firm and in producing the best handling qualities. Overfeeding and crowding too rapidly should in all cases be avoided. Some men are of the opinion that the more they feed the sheep, the better the sheep will do, but this is quite often a mistake. Feeding has its limit, and if fitted so highly that they become soft, or "overdone," sheep will not win in the ring.

It is a pity to see good rams and ewes that are fed so far beyond the limit that they are simply ruined and are worthless for breeding purposes. Such sheep could not even win in the fat classes, as butchers object to a lot of surplus fat on sheep on the block. They should be in nice flesh, but not overfat. The writer himself has been forced more than once to turn down sheep in the ring for this very reason. We often see sheep that are so "blubbery" and overdone that they are unable to stand up long enough in the ring for the judge to pass his decision upon the class in which they are shown. Much improvement must be made in this respect, and showmen must familiarize themselves better with what is called "just in bloom." This condition of bloom is sought by all good judges and should count more for the winning animals than it has in the past.

TRIMMING SHOW SHEEP.

Some writers and farmers have recently taken up arms against sheep trimming. It remains an open question why these men have taken such a step. Has not the shepherd the same right to fix up his stock to make it look best in the show ring as the cattleman, the horseman, and the exhibitor of hogs? Trimming sheep was first put into practice in England. American importers saw the work done in that country and soon followed the example. Nowadays many of the shepherds in this country are men born in England where they have learned this work from their fathers and later have come to America and practice it here.

There is nothing wrong in it. It seems as if only those men who cannot trim their sheep are the ones who protest against this practice. If some one should undertake to stop sheep trimming in England he would be ridiculed, since the English, as a rule, excel in this kind of work and take great pride in bringing a sheep before the judge that is not only well fed, but also carries its best fitted suit of clothes on its body. It does not make much difference to a good judge how well a sheep may be trimmed, as he understands the proper handling of them to find all deficiencies, but it would of course mislead a less experienced man and he ought not to undertake to judge sheep at fairs at all. Trimming sheep is done simply to have them look better when on exhibition, just as men and women wear their best clothes when going to a party.

Trimming sheep should begin just as soon as the wool has grown to such a length that it may be worked upon with the hand shears. The old hand shears, well sharpened and handled by a man who understands his work, will do the task satisfactorily. Two or three trimmings will put the sheep in fine shape. For this purpose, we need a pail of water, a coarse stubble brush to roughen up the wool, and a finer brush with which the wool is wet and brought to the surface. A wet woolen rag is often useful in sponging off the wool to make it fluffy and to free it from dirt which dulls the shears. A halter is also required with which to tie the sheep to a post or fence. Sheep will naturally stand more quietly than lambs. In trimming the animal begin on the top of its shoulder, working backward to the hips and tail. Try to get the back straight. Now the rear end must be trimmed to correspond with the back, and next the left side from the shoulder back to the thigh. The right side comes then, starting from the thigh for-

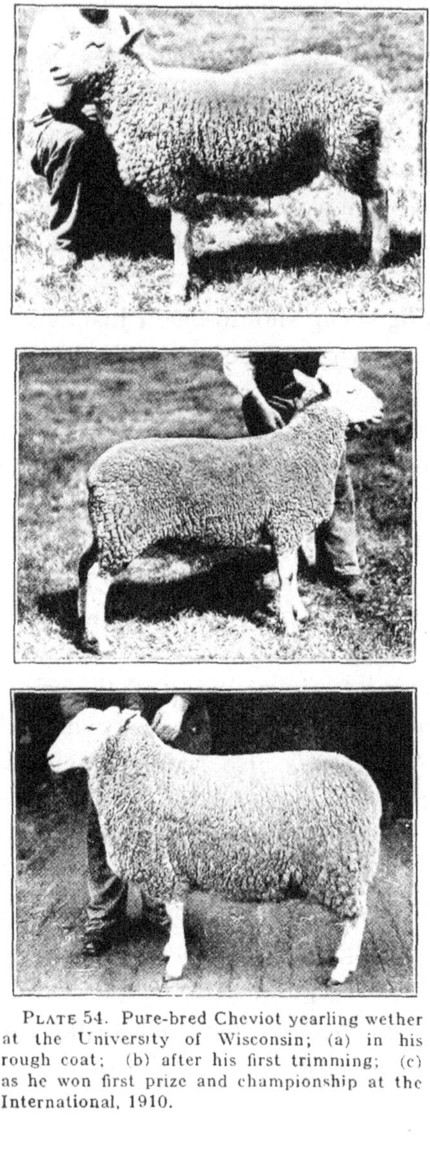

PLATE 54. Pure-bred Cheviot yearling wether at the University of Wisconsin; (a) in his rough coat; (b) after his first trimming; (c) as he won first prize and championship at the International, 1910.

ward. If the operator can use the shears with his left hand he can start on the shoulder and work backward, the same as on the left side. The breast is trimmed next to make the correct lines on that part. Now the left side of the neck is trimmed and then the right side, and finally the neck and head are finished. If a sheep does not have a straight underline some wool may be taken off from the belly.

The first set of illustrations shows a Cheviot yearling wether, first, in his natural rough fleece, second, after the first trimming, and third, when he won first prize and championship at the International in 1910. In the second set are given three similar pictures of an Oxford yearling wether which likewise won first prize and championship at the International in 1910.

To do this work well requires considerable time and a great deal of patience. A person with a sharp eye and a good model in his mind, will make the best trimmer. A systematic way as outlined in the foregoing should be followed in order to perform the work in the best manner. Some people will clip off a little wool at one place and then jump to another place, so that they can never see clearly how much of the work is done and what remains to be done.

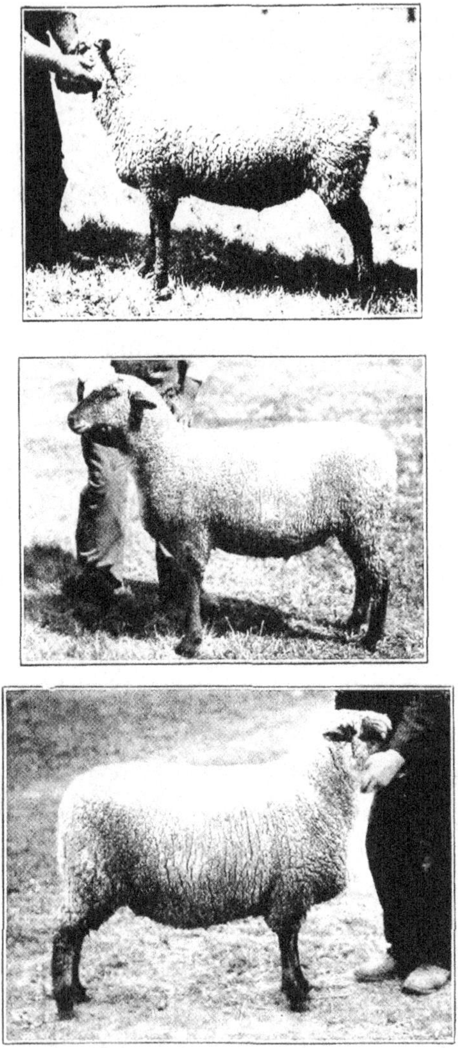

PLATE 55. Pure-bred Oxford yearling wether bred by R. J. Stone, Illinois, and fitted and shown, by the University of Wisconsin; (a) in his rough coat; (b) after his first trimming; (c) as he won first prize and championship at the International 1910.

In the case of Shropshires the covering of wool on their faces and legs counts for a great deal in the show ring. As this wool often becomes clotted together, in fitting the animals it may be necessary to wash it well with warm water, using a woolen rag. Often some sweet oil is used to soften the clotted wool up thoroughly so that it may be combed out with an iron comb. When the wool is then dry it will be fluffy and stand out to the best advantage.

If a show sheep should scour and the wool at its rear become filthy, this filthy wool should not be clipped off with the shears but must be washed out by means of a rag, warm water, and soap. When these locks are clipped off with the shears it gives the sheep a hollow appearance at its twist, while its twist should look full and plump.

A HELP IN SHEEP TRIMMING.

Trimming sheep in hot weather often becomes a difficult task on account of the many flies which annoy the sheep by biting the parts where no wool is growing, such as the face, ears, and legs. The sheep in trying to fight flies shakes its head and stamps its feet constantly, thereby checking the speed of the trimmer, as well as leading him to make false clips or to cut too deeply into the fleece at some places. This trouble can easily be remedied by using a strong solution of any of the coal tar dips, which can be applied to the parts of the sheep which are free from wool, as the ears, face, and legs, with a tin spray pump or by means of a brush. This method relieves the sheep of the annoyance from flies and thus furthers the speed of the trimmer. After being trimmed the sheep should not be allowed to rub itself on sharp corners, posts, nails, or other rough objects.

COLORING SHEEP.

For various reasons show sheep are colored red, yellow, or sometimes brown. The custom of coloring, like trimming, has been introduced into America from England. These various colors on sheep have been the cause of quite a sensation at fairs, and have led men and women to ask whether breeds of sheep naturally grow red, yellow, and brown wool. The writer is decidedly not in favor of the practice. He has never shown a sheep that was colored and never will, because he believes that a sheep with its natural color of wool nicely trimmed looks far better than an animal with a colored fleece.

BLANKETING.

After the sheep have gone through the trimming process and their fleeces look as smooth as a planed board, it is well to cover them with blankets before starting out to the fairs. This will keep the fleeces in good shape, will prevent them from getting roughened up in transit, and will furthermore to a certain extent stop the fingering and spoiling of the appearances of the fleeces by people who thoughtlessly handle the sheep. Blankets, if not adjusted to fit the sheep smoothly, often disfigure it by cutting into the wool at one place or another, especially around the neck of the sheep.

TRAINING SHEEP FOR THE SHOW.

While trimming is being done it is a good idea to have the sheep practice standing right or posing for the judge when in the ring. Many sheep have been found to act very wild and to stand in queer positions in the ring when the judge is to pass on them. On account of their unwieldy conduct and unnatural standing position some prizes have been lost to the owner. If properly handled and given frequent lessons on correct standing they soon learn what is expected of them, and they will not then disappoint their master in the ring at a moment when all little details may bring success or take away prize money from him. Sheep may be trained to follow their master like a dog. Of course, the master must be the one to accomplish these results. As said before, the rough, coarse, and brutal fellow will never get a sheep to do anything for him, as it remembers only too well the kind of treatment it has received.

SHELTER FOR SHOW SHEEP.

When fitting has begun great care must be taken that the show sheep do not get wet. If a clean fleece is desired, the sheep should be washed thoroughly at the time when fitting begins. From then on by no means should they be allowed to become wet. During the fitting period the yolk distributes itself nicely throughout the fleece, and if the sheep is exposed to a heavy rain the yolk will be washed out, which destroys the lustre and bright, healthy appearance. When the fleece has once been spoiled somewhat, especially when it has already been trimmed once or twice, it can never be made right again. While it has been stated that sheep should be turned out on pasture nights to get lots of exercise, it should be borne in mind that we do not mean on nights when rain is expected or predicted. The writer recalls many a night when he turned out his show sheep, not expecting that it would rain before the next morning. A heavy thunder shower would come up after midnight and wake him out of his sleep. As quickly as possible he would then run to the place where the sheep were kept and get them under roof before they got wet, although he himself was perhaps wet to the skin on returning home. This, however, made no difference to him for he rejoiced if he succeeded in keeping his show sheep dry. This, fellow sheepmen, is one of the numerous self-sacrifices mentioned before.

TRIMMING THE FEET OF SHOW SHEEP.

It has been advised in this work that sheep should have their feet trimmed and looked after at least twice a year, in spring and fall, but sheep being fitted for shows need to have their feet trimmed much more frequently. These sheep are more or less confined and do not wear down their hoofs as much as sheep that are constantly out of doors in the summer months. Furthermore, from observation it seems that when a sheep is fed well and is putting on flesh its hoofs grow in proportion to the amount of flesh put on its body. Therefore, to keep them straight on their feet the wise shepherd examines them once every month and removes all surplus hoof.

REDUCING SHOW SHEEP AFTER FAIRS.

When sheep have been once highly fitted and shown they cannot be kept in that condition, but have to be reduced in flesh. For instance, a winning yearling will not be a winner the following year as a two-year-old, unless some of the old flesh has been taken off and new flesh substituted in its place. The old flesh left on the sheep becomes soft and stale, and the skin gets pale and will not have the desired "bloom."

This work of reducing flesh has to be done just as carefully as putting on flesh. The writer knows of a first prize winning sheep that was sold to a man who did not know how to reduce it. In spite of the fact that he was warned to be careful and not let it down in condition too fast, he killed the sheep in less than one month by reducing the flesh too quickly through cutting down the feed. The reduction in feed, especially grain, must be made very gradually, so that the sheep do not experience a great drop in the amount of feed at any time. Remember that lots of exercise is necessary to bring show sheep back into natural condition, just as much as it was in fitting them for the ring. Indeed, exercise is one of the most important factors in letting them down in condition.

CHAPTER X.

FITTING WETHERS FOR SHOWS.

The work of so fitting and preparing wethers for fat stock shows that they will win on the hoof as well as on the block may be considerd the most difficult task of all show fitting. In the breeding classes the sheep are only passed upon when alive, while in the fat classes they are first judged alive and are then sent to the slaughter house where the expert butcher and cutter determines the final merit of the carcasses. The material contained in this book is not based upon reading agricultural papers and it is not taken from books or the experience of others, but is based upon the practical experience and knowledge gained by the author in fitting many wethers which have won first prizes, championships and grand championships on the hoof, as well as on the block.

A great many of the show sheep in the breeding classes at state fairs and other large shows are imported from England, where they have received part or all of their fitting from the English shepherds before coming to this country. It is an easy matter for the Americans to keep them in the trim to which the English have brought them. For-

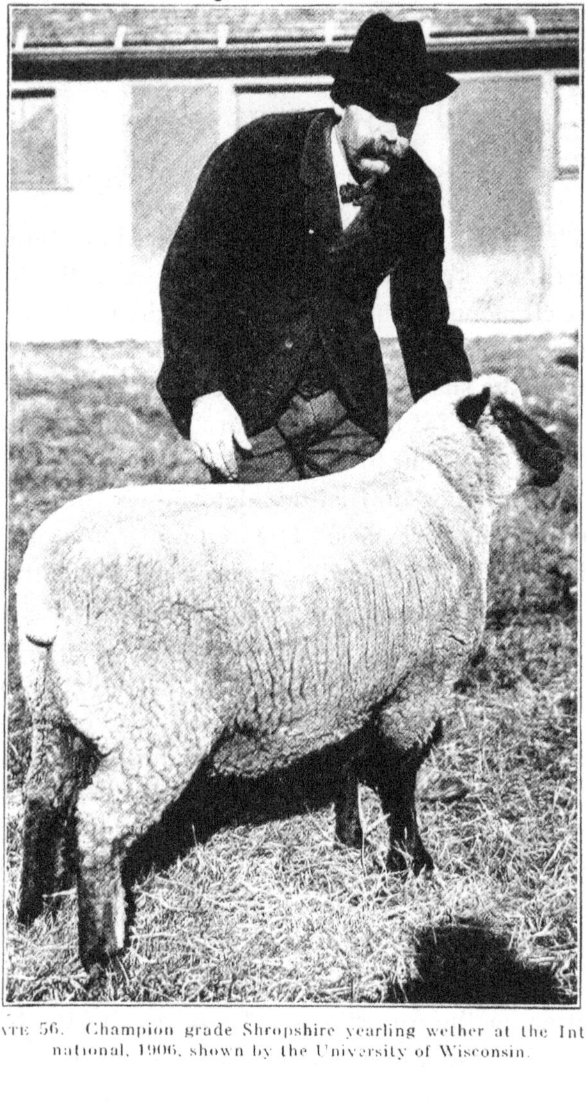

PLATE 56. Champion grade Shropshire yearling wether at the International, 1906, shown by the University of Wisconsin.

merly, only once in a while were a few fat wethers imported from England, and it was therefore left to the shepherds of this country to fit and prepare the candidates in this class of sheep for our fat stock shows. During recent years, however, the American fitter has been compelled to stand face to face in the fat stock show ring with his English and Canadian brothers, who have brought their home-fitted wethers directly from their native country to the International Live Stock Show and other fat stock shows. It can easily be understood what a struggle it must be to compete with an English fitter, considering the climatic condtions and other advantages which the English have over the Americans. Therefore, the American who succeeds in defeating the imported English stock has won a great victory.

Type, fleece, and color of skin are not as essential in the show ring for fat wethers as for sheep of the breeding classes, because there are other factors of still greater importance for sheep to go on the block. In the fat wether on the hoof his form and the amount and kind of flesh he carries are the most important points. When on the block the most essential points of the carcass are the percentage of edible meat, and the quality, color, and marbling of the meat. There are three distinct classes of wethers. The first class is not far enough advanced in condition and flesh, the second is just right, and the third is too far advanced. The second or middle class is of course the one which is successful.

Thorough knowledge and great judgment in feeding are required to get the animal in just the proper condition. In late years judges of fat wethers have been far more accurate in making their decisions than they were in former years. They know that the expert carcass judge next passes his judgment upon the animals and brings to light either the correctness or incorrectness of the decision when on foot. To fit a wether with the highest quality of meat, so that every part of his body is covered smoothly with the firmest kind of flesh, and so that his carcass does not show any surplus fat, or tallow, and yet possesses a mellow touch, is by no means a small task.

SELECTION OF WETHERS.

As in the case of breeding sheep, only well-balanced animals should be selected to fit for the fat stock ring. Wethers that have long legs, crooked feet, or broken-down pasterns are of no use. The right kind of wether should have an even, straight, smooth, broad back and should be free from coarseness in any part. While we like to see as much type as possible, still it is far less important in fat wethers than in breeding animals. In picking out a wether to fit for the fat class the most importance should be placed on his conformation,

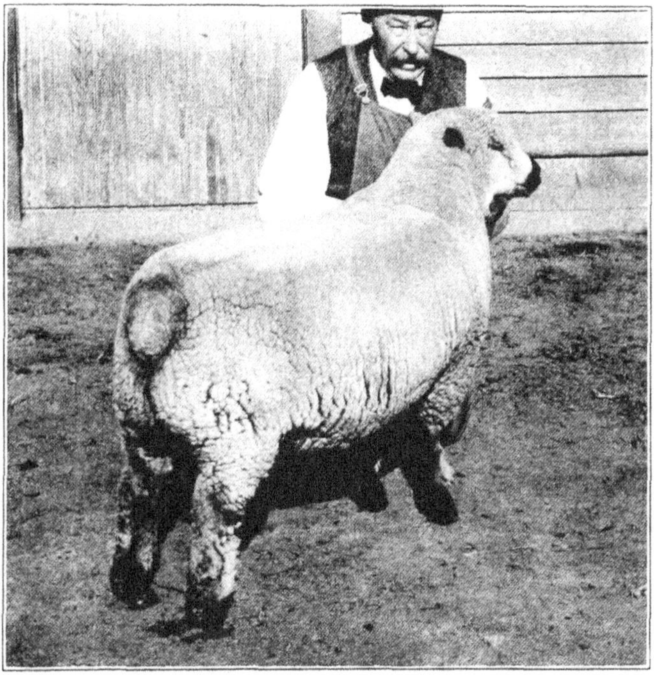

PLATE 57. Pure-bred Shropshire yearling wether. First prize and champion at the International, 1917. Shown by the University of Wisconsin.

firm handling qualities, and density of fleece. In the writer's experience no wether which has had a long, loose, open fleece, for his particular breed has ever proved to be a prize winner when fattened. His favorites have always been those with comparatively short and very dense fleeces. If a wether handles soft at the start he will be much worse at the end of the fitting period, and no soft, blubbery wether can win if a capable judge is making the awards.

SHEARING WETHERS.

Wethers for show can be sheared much later in the season than breeding animals, since the length of the wool does not count for much on wethers in the show ring. Wethers which have been sheared too early suffer a great deal on hot summer days and do not progress nearly so well as when sheared later on, although judgment must be used not to go to an extreme and let them suffer from heat with their old, long coats on. A short fleece tends to make them more firm and solid, while a long fleece makes them seem soft. Wethers that are brought into the show ring with comparatively short fleeces on them generally handle well, and these good handlers are selected as winners.

AGE TO SHOW WETHERS.

In earlier years fat wethers, at least at some shows, consisted of three classes, two-year-olds, yearlings, and lambs. Nowadays the two-year-old class is not listed, and the writer believes that in time the yearling class will also drop out of existence. The nice juicy lamb chop is in just as great demand at the present time as baby beef. The American people desire the youngest and juiciest kind of meat for consumption, and they find the lamb better than the yearling. It may be said right here that only an extra good lamb should be carried over to be fitted as a yearling. Unless one can foresee that the lamb will be a prize winner as a yearling there is no use feeding it another year, since the lamb will sell for about as much as the yearling, and one year's feed is saved.

BEST CLASS TO FIT

If the writer had a choice in selecting yearlings to be fitted from a lot which contained some that had been fitted and shown as lambs and others that had not been fitted previously, both lots being equally good in general make-up, he would immediately decide upon those that had not been fitted and shown as lambs. He would do this because it is very difficult to make a prize winning lamb a prize winning yearling. Yet in one instance the writer was very fortunate in taking first, championship, and grand championship prizes at the International Live Stock Show at Chicago on a yearling which the previous year, as a lamb, had won first prize. However, this was a very exceptional case. Sheep with new flesh and in new bloom are the best kind to show.

FEEDING THE WETHERS.

It takes from four to four and one-half months of steady feeding to get yearling wethers in proper shape for the show ring and the block. Of course animals in a rather thin condition will require an even longer feeding period. This work should never be hurried and crowded along too rapidly, for if the wethers are pushed along too fast the chances are that they will become soft and lose their firm handling quality. Lambs, however, are brought right forward from the day they commence eating. It is very essential that lambs and yearlings should not be overheated, which often happens in hot weather. Therefore, especially during the hot weather, grain should be fed but once a day, until cooler weather comes on towards fall. Cabbage and turnips tend to keep them cool when fed to them during the warmest weather. When there is a shortage of pasture clover or alfalfa hay may be fed.

THE BEST GRAIN MIXTURE TO FEED.

In the writer's experience no better results have been obtained in producing winners on the hoof, as well as on the block, than by feeding yearling wethers a grain mixture consisting of one part bran, two parts oats, one part cracked field peas, and one part barley. A *little* corn may be added in place of peas, if these are not available. Heavy corn feeding, however, should be avoided, as it

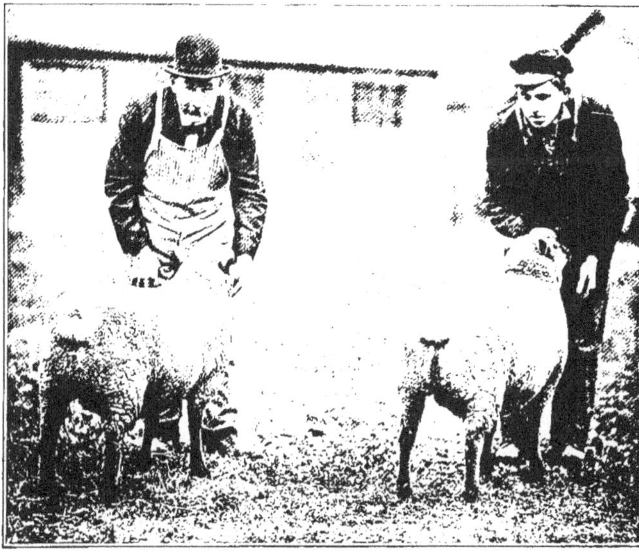

PLATE 58. A pair of prize-winning Southdown yearling wethers shown by the University of Wisconsin.

produces too soft a carcass, which does not insure firm handling when alive and shows surplus fat when dressed. Many fitters of wethers have learned bitter lessons from feeding too much corn.

This rich grain ration will not do for lambs in warm weather, for it is too heavy. During the warm weather a mixture of bran, oats, and a very little oilmeal has given satisfaction for feeding lambs. In cool weather a few peas and a little barley or corn will not injure the lambs, but, in general, lambs need very close watching so as not to overload them with grain, which causes overheating and foundering. They should, however, have all the green feeds they can eat. During the hottest months of the fitting period the best feeds for them are cabbage, rape, green clover, turnips, or rutabagas. At this time these feeds, together with some good clover or alfalfa hay, preferably the latter, should be their main ration. The feeder must judge as to the amount of grain to be fed to each animal.

Often the writer has been feeding yearlings heavily for two or three weeks, because he thought that they were not advancing rapidly. After handling them again, he found that they were gaining too fast, and therefore the grain ration was decreased somewhat so that at show time they would be in just the proper condition. The touch of the feeder's hand must guide the feeding Lambs hardly ever get too fat.

FITTING YEARLING WETHERS.

The writer will now give the course pursued by him in fitting yearling wethers and lambs that have been successfully shown at the largest fat stock shows.

All the animals which have been fitted for these shows have been fed experimentally on different rations in order to study the value of various feeds. In so doing all the feed except pasturage is weighed and recorded, enabling the writer to give here the most successful rations.

The yearlings are sheared from April 30 to May 10, according to the weather. They are turned out on grass about May 20. No grain, hay, or other feed is now given them. About July 10 they are brought to the barn, and from this date a small allowance of grain is fed every morning, after which they are driven into a small pasture near the barn where there are nice shade trees.

About July 15 the first trimming or so-called blocking-out is done. A cool day should always be chosen for trimming any sheep, as otherwise they are apt to become overheated from struggling before they become accustomed to being trimmed. About August 10 the pasture is generally becoming scant and some nice clover hay is therefore fed to them in the evening. At the same time the early cabbage is ready for feeding, and each wether receives from one and one-half to two pounds per head daily.

About August 15 they are trimmed the second time, and where the wool was too short at the time of the first trimming to give the wether the proper shape, it is now trimmed to the best form possible. The grain ration is also increased a little at this

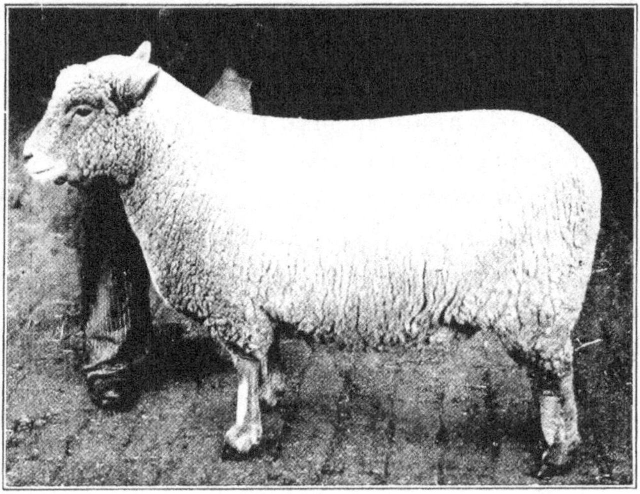

PLATE 59. Pure-bred Southdown yearling wether winning third prize in open class and championship in college class at the International, 1910, shown by the University of Wisconsin.

time. Beginning September 20, grain is fed twice daily, the full amount formerly fed being still given in the morning, but only a little being at first given in the evening. The amount is gradually increased as the weather gets cooler. A little hay is now fed in the morning after the grain is given and before they go out to pasture. The wethers now receive a third trimming, after which they need only be kept smooth, as their form has been shaped at previous trimmings. At each trimming the wethers are carefully handled and their condition studied, so that their grain ration may be increased or decreased in view of the time when they are to be shown. About October 1 rutabagas are ready to be fed, and as excessive cabbage feeding may tend to make the wethers a little soft in handling, each wether receives about two pounds of rutabagas each day chopped up with a root cutter. The amount of cabbage is reduced at this time to one pound for each wether, making two pounds of roots and one pound of cabbage for each wether daily.

This ration is continued until November 1 when cabbage is abandoned and the same amount of roots, two pounds, still fed. The aim from this time on is to feed them mostly on grain and hay, so that they will become firm and hard and be solid in handling, which is the main point in the ring as well as on the block. If time permits they are given another trimming about the middle of October. About November 15 they are touched up with the shears for the last time and are then covered with blankets.

Their feet receive careful attention at least every five or six weeks, and the hoofs are trimmed when found necessary. Until November 1 the wethers are out of doors every day, with the exception of rainy days, principally to get all the exercise pos-

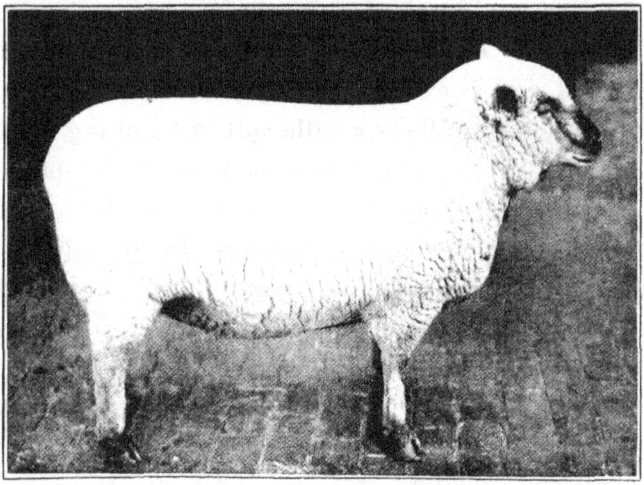

Plate 60. Grand champion pure-bred Southdown yearling wether at the International, 1910, shown by the Huntleywood Farm, Quebec, Canada.

sible. After November 1 they are kept in the barn day and night, and only in the nicest weather are they allowed to run about in the sheep yard for a couple of hours at a time. For shows that are held earlier in the fall than the International the feeding has to be crowded along a little more. Before loading on the car for shipment to the show they are fed only a half meal of dry feed, to prevent scouring.

When feeding yearling wethers and lambs we often find that some of them become troubled with sore sheaths. These should be treated as already stated elsewhere in this work. They should be washed out with a syringe a few times, using one quart of warm water to one-half teaspoonful of permanganate of potash, and a little iodoform should be sprinkled on the sore. This treatment will soon remedy the trouble.

FITTING WETHER LAMBS.

Lambs that are to be shown late in the fall are generally put into the barn about September 1. Their grain ration has been outlined before. During warm weather they should be fed all the green feed they will eat, such as cabbage, roots, and green clover. Care must be taken that they are not overheated and foundered from too heavy grain feeding. There is, however, no danger of getting lambs too fat through heavy grain feeding, for they are growing too rapidly to put on much fat. In cooler weather more grain may safely be fed, and the allowance of green feed cut down somewhat, for feeding an excessive amount of green feed continuously is apt to make the lambs a little soft. Of course, there is not nearly so much danger of lambs handling soft as there is in the case of yearlings. If a lamb at any time becomes overheated and founders from eating too much grain, it should be separated from the rest of the

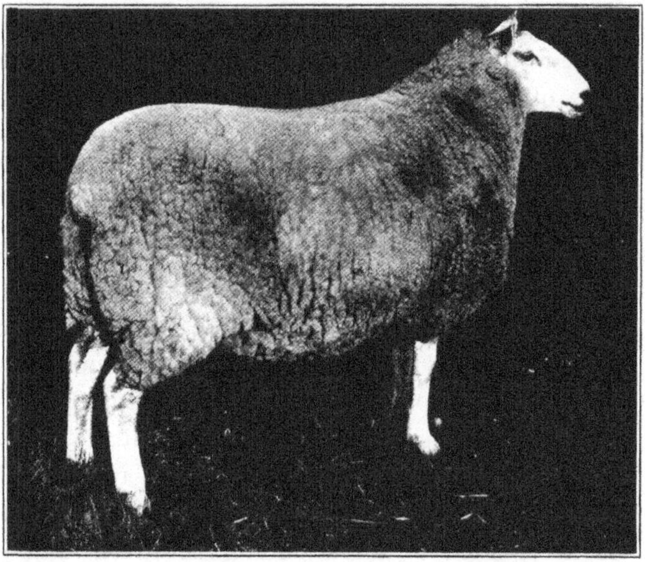

PLATE 61. Champion pure-bred Cheviot yearling wether at the International, 1909, shown by the University of Wisconsin.

flock and be given a dose of two tablespoonfuls of epsom salts dissolved in water for a physic. If this does not bring about the desired results the dose should be repeated. The lamb should not be given any more grain until the trouble is over. When lambs are overheated they are stiff in their legs and body, shake when walking, and drink lots of water. If they are once foundered it is difficult to get them right again.

SYMPTOMS OF FOUNDER.

The term foundering is well known to many expert show fitters. It does not make any difference how well any man is posted in fitting sheep, he will once in a while have a foundered lamb. In a bunch of eight to ten head fed in the most careful manner, there are perhaps one or two which are more greedy than the others. By this greediness they get a little more grain than their share, and if the grain is of a heavy, rich nature during warm weather they become foundered.

A foundered lamb becomes stiff on all its four legs. It walks just as if it did not have any joints in its limbs, its temperature is abnormally high, and its breathing is very fast, indicating a feverish condition. It does not care to walk even a short distance and lies down every twenty to thirty feet, and sometimes oftener, when it is driven. This condition is due to an overheated, so-called "burned out" stomach caused by eating too much heavy grain. While a certain amount of grain may bring on this trouble in hot weather, in cooler weather this same amount, or even more, would not hurt the lamb in the least.

REMEDY FOR FOUNDER.

A foundered lamb should be removed from the rest and placed in as cool quarters as can be given it. The grain allowance should be discontinued,

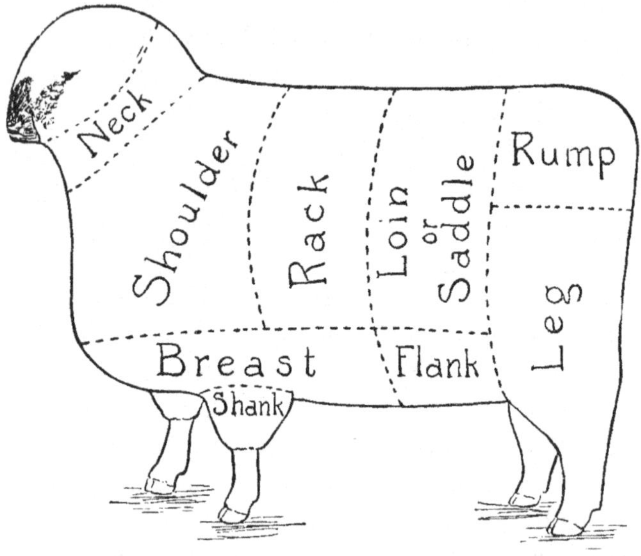

PLATE 62. The outline of a sheep showing the location of the various butcher's cuts.

and it should be fed on green feeds, such as rape, cabbage, turnips, and green clover, with perhaps a little good hay. The lamb should remain in these cool quarters until the feverish condition has disappeared. While there is scarcely any medicine that will help the lamb so affected, yet a quar-

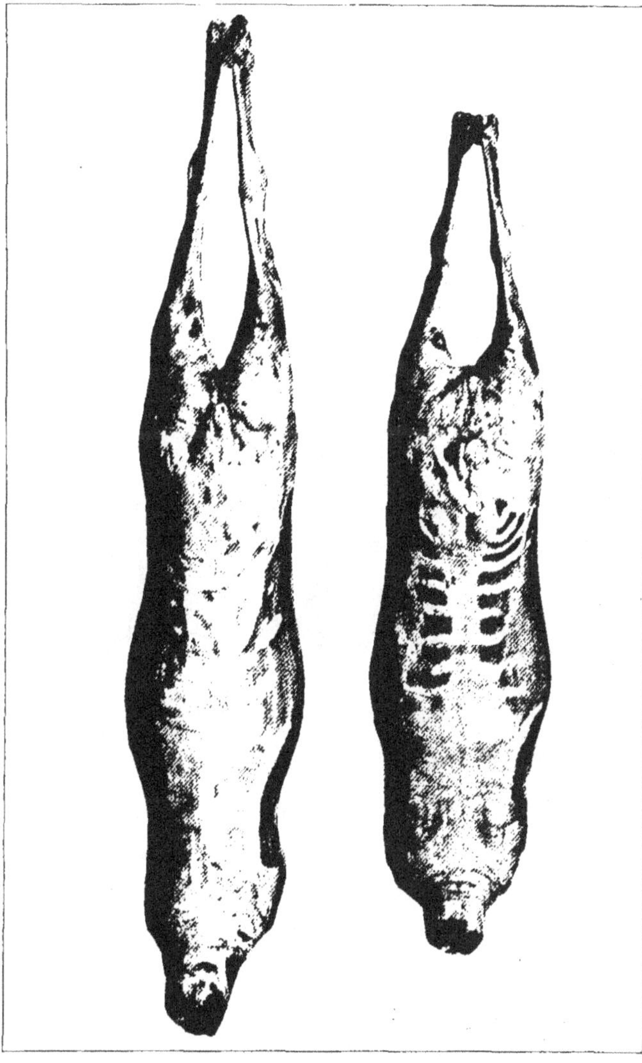

PLATE 63. Two lamb carcasses. The one at the left is the kind sought by the butcher. It has the most valuable cuts. Note the shortness of neck, width of back and loin, full hind quarter, and short legs, as compared with the one at the right.

ter of a teaspoonful of saltpeter given twice a day in a little water may prove of some help. A dose or two of physic is also beneficial.

TRIMMING THE LAMBS.

Lambs do not necessarily need to be trimmed until they are brought to the barn, which, as already mentioned, is about September 1. On any

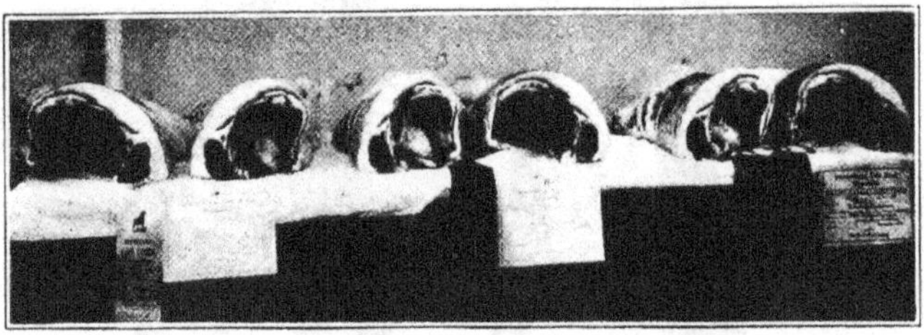

PLATE 64. Dressed carcasses of yearling wethers, first, second, and third prize winners. All three were Southdowns shown by the University of Wisconsin at the International of 1913. The one on the right was the champion carcass of the show

cool day after that date they may receive their first trimming. Three trimmings should bring them into very nice form, as their wool is longer than that on yearlings, and therefore they can be blocked out with fewer trimmings. While they are being fitted it is necessary to give their feet attention, one or two trimmings usually being necessary to keep their hoofs in proper shape.

SELECTING BLOCK WINNERS.

Very often many of the prize winning wethers on the hoof do not win on the block. This is probably true in more cases in England than in America. At the English shows fatter, softer, and more blubbery wethers are shown than in America, and these animals are awarded the prize money be-

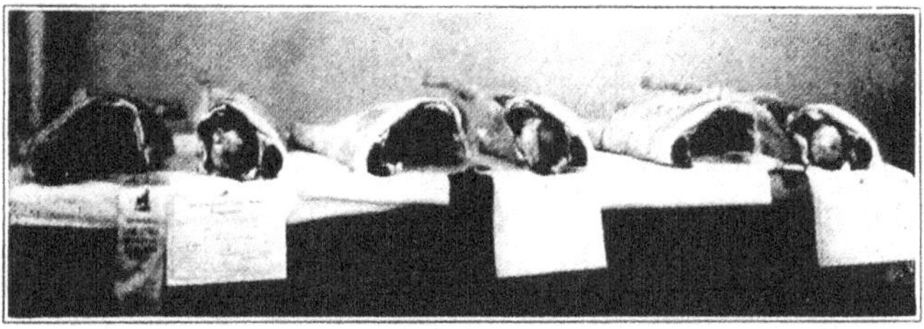

PLATE 65. Dressed carcasses of lambs, first, second, and third prize winners. All three were Southdowns. The second and third prize winners were shown by the University of Wisconsin at the International of 1913.

cause the English seem to like fatter mutton than do Americans. The American judges of fat wethers have come to realize what it is that the butcher wants when the animal is brought on the block.

It has been demonstrated time and again that the Southdown excels all other breeds when it comes to the block test. This breed of sheep more adequately fills the requirements of what constitutes a good form, and shows the proper mixing of fat with lean meat, which forms what is termed "nicely marbled" meat. The carcass possesses great thickness, and has the least tallow in proportion to the lean meat. The Shropshire stands next in rank to the Southdown, judging from the winnings by this breed at the International during the past fourteen years.

A person who has carefully observed the awards made in the carcass classes, can pretty well judge when the sheep are alive which of them will win on the block. Such carcasses will win that cut the most edible meat, especially those parts that sell for the highest prices, providing, of course, that the meat is of the proper quality. A wether that usually wins on the block is of the following description when alive. To start with he has a very short neck, is broad and smooth on the shoulders, with a well-developed back, has no depression between shoulder and first rib, and has sides which do not bulge out. His back is very smooth and broad, being especially broad and thick over the loin, with a long, wide hind quarter filled out well in the twist nearly to the hocks. There is no surplus fat on the tail-head, nor on the fore flank, the belly does not hang down too deep, and the legs are short and not coarse in bone. The wether must have a very firm handling quality, as those that handle soft alive will also handle soft when dressed. If fed on the right kind of feed the carcass will display the desired so-called "cream" color.

The writer has fitted the champion carcass prize winners ten years out of fourteen years' showing at the International, and has won many other prizes in these classes. He has therefore gained some knowledge, at least, in this line of work. At the close of this discussion it may be stated that a wether that has the right conformation and is fed the proper quantity of the right kind of feed is bound to win on the block. Among these feeds, alfalfa and clover hay, oats, barley, bran, and especially peas may be highly recommended.

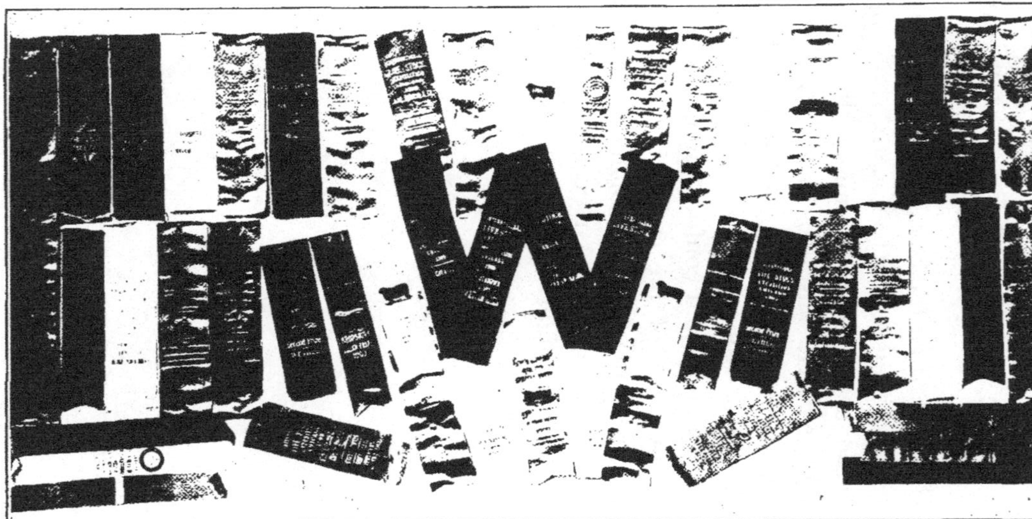

PLATE 66. The Sheperd's reward. Ribbons representing careful selection, faithful, painstaking labor, and proper judgment in feeding. Won by the University of Wisconsin at the International, 1909.

CHAPTER XI.

THE ART AND METHOD OF JUDGING SHEEP.

JUDGING SHEEP AT FAIRS, IN THE CLASSROOM, OR ON THE FARM.

Acting as the judge of sheep at fairs is by no means a small task, for the person who performs this duty assumes a large measure of responsibility. Incompetence of a judge is inexcusable in every event. No person should ever attempt to act as judge, even at a county fair, unless he possesses the necessary qualifications. Wherever judging is done at any fair, whether large or small, a crowd of interested onlookers watch the work and decisions of the judge, and aim to learn the highest type and conformation of animals. If the judge is not capable of selecting the best animals for the prize winners from those which are brought before him, but selects unworthy candidates, he is not only depriving exhibitors of their prize money and the honor rightfully belonging to them, but he is also deceiving the interested onlookers. He conveys the wrong impression of what constitutes the highest class of well-conditioned show animals to those who come to the fair to learn. Any person guilty of awarding prizes to unworthy animals is committing an offense which he cannot rectify later on. Generally the practical sheepmen who are themselves good breeders and successful exhibitors have given the best satisfaction as judges. It is clear to everyone that a man who for years has cared for and raised sheep and is familiar with show yard deceptions will make a more efficient judge than one who only occasionally sees a sheep.

The judge must possess the following qualifications before he is competent to officiate in the ring:

First, he must be thoroughly familiar with the standard of excellence of each individual breed of sheep he is to pass upon.

Second, he must have learned the practical manner of handling and examining sheep.

Third, he must possess the indispensable sharpness to quickly see the best points in one sheep and the defective ones in another.

Fourth, when questioned he must be able to state the reasons upon which he bases his decision.

Fifth, he should be able to pass judgment on a class in a fairly speedy manner.

Sixth, and most important of all, the judge must be strictly honest.

In the show ring he should accord the same treatment to his enemy that he does to his friend. Absolute impartiality should govern his decision. Of course no judge can please all exhibitors, as the better animals will win and the inferior ones will always lose. But if a judge who understands his business gives all concerned a square deal, not much criticism will follow his work. The judge who has rated the animals correctly can leave the fair grounds with a clear conscience and with a feeling that he has accorded justice to all. Difference of opinion will always prevail, but on the whole general satisfaction attends the decisions of the capable judge.

A thorough knowledge of how to judge sheep is highly important not only for the student and for one who intends to judge at fairs, but also for every sheep raiser. In the selection of breeding rams and ewes for his flock, the sheep raiser will be less likely to make mistakes, if he has a clear idea of the best types and forms of sheep. A flock owner often has several well-formed, well-built sheep in the flock but fails to detect them because he is unable to recognize the best types and forms. A great variation is often seen in sheep of the same breed so that it is essential that one be well-informed about all the fine points in order to make intelligent selections. This is true whether one is a judge at fairs, a breeder of sheep, or a student in an agricultural college. To know how to judge sheep will aid materially in the upbuilding of sheep husbandry in general, besides creating a desire to raise the better and more profitable kind in preference to the inferior grades.

FEW FITTED TO JUDGE.

Today we have not a great many judges of sheep in America who have attained a national reputation in this line of work. The number of these is so small that they can almost be counted on a man's ten fingers. The majority of them are men who are quite advanced in age, and their years in life are counted. Therefore it is to be hoped that more young men who like sheep will take an interest in this work and become competent sheep judges. They are surely needed to follow the footsteps of the old veterans.

Some men do not make an attempt to judge sheep, in spite of the fact that they could easily fit themselves to do so. The simple reason for this is, perhaps, that they are afraid that they cannot come up to the master shepherd's work with the shears in trimming, for judging is somewhat difficult for a man who himself is not a practical shepherd and has never fitted or trimmed a sheep.

A good judge must necessarily have the proper type and conformation of each breed of sheep strongly fixed in his mind, and must know the right way to handle sheep, in order to judge sheep satisfactorily. It should be remembered at all times that in judging breeding classes, one must hold strongly to breed type; while in judging fat sheep, less attention is paid to type, wool, skin, and color of face or legs, and more to the form of the sheep, its proper meatiness, and the best development of those parts which will bring the highest price on the butcher's block. However, fat sheep must also possess some type of their respective breeds.

GENERAL DIRECTIONS FOR JUDGING.

The method given should be followed at all times, except in the case of sheep which are permitted to have horns, when one does not need to examine the poll of the head; or in the case of fat sheep, when one does not need to look at the length or quality of the wool, or for the color of the skin. All other points are practically the same in both breeding and fat classes.

The age of the sheep must be determined first of all, so that no exhibitor shows a sheep which is older or younger than the class in which it belongs. Age is a very important point. The writer has judged thousands of sheep at many different county and state fairs, national and international shows, and has many times found sheep that were

THE UNIVERSITY OF WISCONSIN,

SCORE CARD FOR

MUTTON SHEEP.

SCALE OF POINTS	Possible Score	Points Deficient: Student's Score	Points Deficient: Corrected.
Age............................**Teeth**....................			
GENERAL APPEARANCE—24 POINTS			
Weight...........estimated...............actual pounds according to age......................	6		
Form, low, long, symmetrical, compact, and evenly covered with firm flesh........	10		
Quality, clean bone; silky hair..............	6		
Temperament..	2		
HEAD AND NECK—9 POINTS			
Muzzle, fair size; nostrils large; lips thin; mouth large..................................	2		
Eyes, full; bright....................................	1		
Face, short, bold expression..................	1		
Forehead, broad	1		
Ears, fine, erect..	1		
Neck, thick, short; throat clean............	3		
FOREQUARTERS—13 POINTS			
Shoulder Vein, full..................................	2		
Shoulders, covered, compact.................	3		
Chest, deep, wide, large girth..................	3		
Brisket, full prominent; breast wide.. ..	2		
Legs, straight, short, wide apart, strong; forearm full, shank smooth................	3		
BODY—13 POINTS			
Back, straight, wide	4		
Loin, broad, thick.....................................	4		
Ribs, deep, arched...................................	3		
Flank, low, thick, making underline straight..	2		
HINDQUARTERS—17 POINTS			
Hips, smooth, far apart...........................	3		
Rump, long, level, wide..........................	4		
Thighs, full, well fleshed..	3		
Twist, plump, deep..................................	4		
Legs, straight, short, strong, shank smooth...	3		
CONSTITUTION—10 POINTS			
Girth, large...	3		
Skin, pink color..	3		
Fleece, dense and even over body, yolk abundant..	4		
WOOL—14 POINTS			
Quantity, long, dense, even....................	6		
Quality, fine, soft, pure, even.........	4		
Condition, bright, strong, clean...........	4		
Total..	100		

exhibited in wrong age classes. In some cases, exhibitors have done this to try out the judge to see if he knew his business. It is also necessary to make sure that each sheep shown in a class belongs to the sex that the class calls for. The writer has found cases where ram lambs were shown in ewe lamb classes, and wethers in ram classes. All of these points should not be overlooked, as they are of great importance.

It is also a good plan to let the sheep walk around the show ring before making a decision, in order to see that none are lame in one foot or leg. This often cannot be discovered, for some shepherds know how to hold a sheep in the ring so as to hide this defect. Style and carriage, as well as active movement, should also be considered when the sheep is turned loose in the ring. This method is often very helpful when there is close competition. For instance, a very fat, overdone, sluggish ram or ewe should never be placed over one which is in the pink of condition, and full of life and vigor, provided the latter has no other serious faults or defects. To make sure of these points, the judge is almost obliged to turn the sheep loose in the ring. Serious cases of lameness often disqualify sheep from competition. However, good judgment must be exercised to ascertain whether the injury is permanent or only temporary.

JUDGING RAM CLASSES.

In passing judgment on classes of rams, it is also important for the judge to examine the scrotum of each, to find out whether or not the ram is fully developed. In cases where the ram has only one testicle instead of two, he should be disqualified on this account. This is important, for the writer has found many rams in show rings that had this defect, and a judge is liable to severe criticism if he overlooks anything of this sort. In selecting a ram to head the flock, an examination of the scrotum should not be forgotten.

The judging of sheep in general is perhaps more difficult than that of other classes of stock, because the wool hides many defects which can only be found by the proper methods of handling. Nevertheless, if a man is once accustomed to this work and knows the proper method of handling, he will not make many blunders in judging the largest classes at any fair, whether county, state, national or international.

For the benefit of the student in agriculture who takes up work in sheep husbandry and for every other person who wants to learn sheep judging, the writer will show in the accompanying illustrations, the most helpful, up-to-date methods of examining sheep so that none of the important points are overlooked. The latest standards given by the respective associations are also included. No time or money has been spared in securing photographs of the different breeds of sheep which show the most typical up-to-date types and characteristics of the different breeds.

PROPER METHOD OF HANDLING SHEEP IN JUDGING.

In judging sheep, the eye should be trained in such a way that it will detect any deficiencies in a sheep by a single glance. It is therefore advisable to look at a sheep first, before putting the hands on it. After the judge has observed the breed characteristics, the general form of the body, the kind of wool, the build of the legs and the size of the bone, he will have a pretty good idea of the rank of the sheep. Then by the use of his hands, he will find all other defects which may be hidden beneath the covering of wool. It is advisable while the body is being handled, that the judge keep all his fingers on both hands close together so as not to mar the evenness and smoothness of the fleece.

EXAMINING THE HEAD AND DETERMINING THE AGE.

In judging rams, one should examine the head closely, as it should be broader and show more masculinity than that of the ewe. A short, broad, masculine head, with bold eyes, indicates a sire

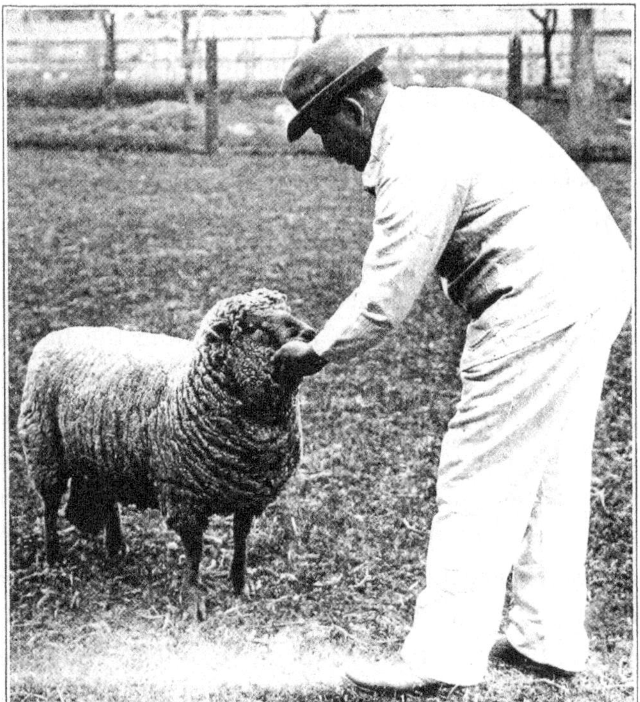

PLATE 67. Ram, looking at the head and eyes. The shape of the head, the masculinity, and the color of the face should be observed

of vigor and prepotency. The color of the face of both ram and ewe and the covering of wool must be in compliance with the standard of each individual breed. When examining the head, first of all, the age of the sheep in the ring should be determined, and if there is one that is older or younger than the class calls for, it must be disregarded. The method of determining the age is shown on page 31. The quality of the sheep may also be noted at this time by either the fine and silky or the coarse hair growing on the sheep's nose.

WATCH FOR HORNS OR A GOITRE.

In judging sheep, especially rams of the breeds which should be free from horns or stubs of horns, the judge may easily determine this fact by placing two fingers of the right hand on the poll of the head as shown in Figure 68. Often these stubs of horns are hidden in the wool which has grown over them so that they are not visible to the eye. Stubs are seldom found on ewes. By placing the left hand on the sheep's throat it may be determined whether the sheep has a goitre. If the ram or ewe is found to have a noticeable goitre, the sheep may be disqualified. It is a serious matter to use a ram or ewe for breeding that has such a

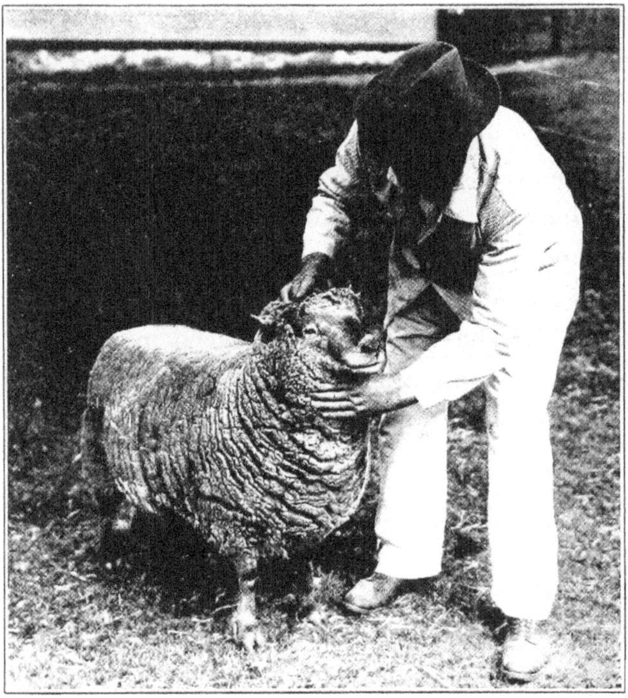

PLATE 68. Finding with two fingers of the right hand whether the sheep is free from stubs of horns, with the left whether it is free from a goitre.

defect, for it is very difficult to raise the offspring. In many cases this defect is inherited. In judging fat sheep, however, a goitre would not be as objectionable.

EXAMINING THE THICKNESS AND LENGTH OF NECK.

In the foregoing, it has been stated that it is very essential that a good sheep have a broad head.

When this is the case, the sheep usually has a thick, short neck. On a ram, of course, we expect to find a thicker neck than on a ewe, but on the ewe while her feminine character allows her to have a neck that is not as thick as that of a ram, it must be short. When a sheep has a short, thick neck, it adds greatly to its appearance; and if found on a ram, one can generally rely upon his being a good sire. Furthermore, the meat cut from the neck is of the cheaper kind as compared to the other parts, and if the butcher has bought the

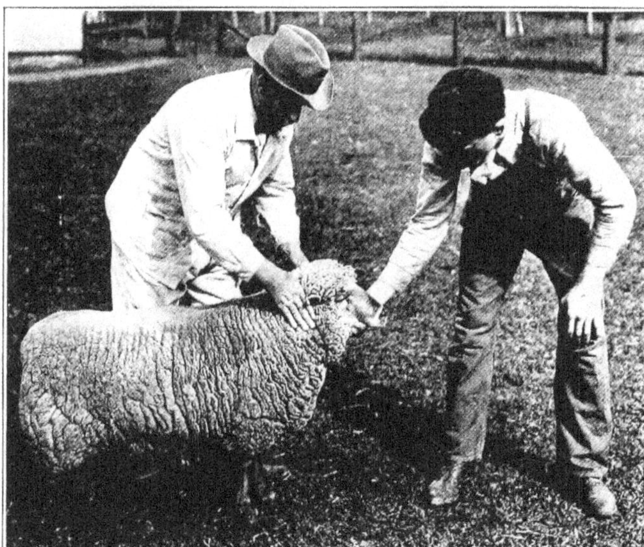

PLATE 69. Determining the thickness of the neck. The neck should be thick and short, especially on the ram.

sheep by the pound and has very much of this to sell, it becomes a loss to him. The larger breeds naturally have longer necks than the smaller ones, but every flock-owner of any breed should aim to breed a sheep with a short neck, since this is the kind the market demands.

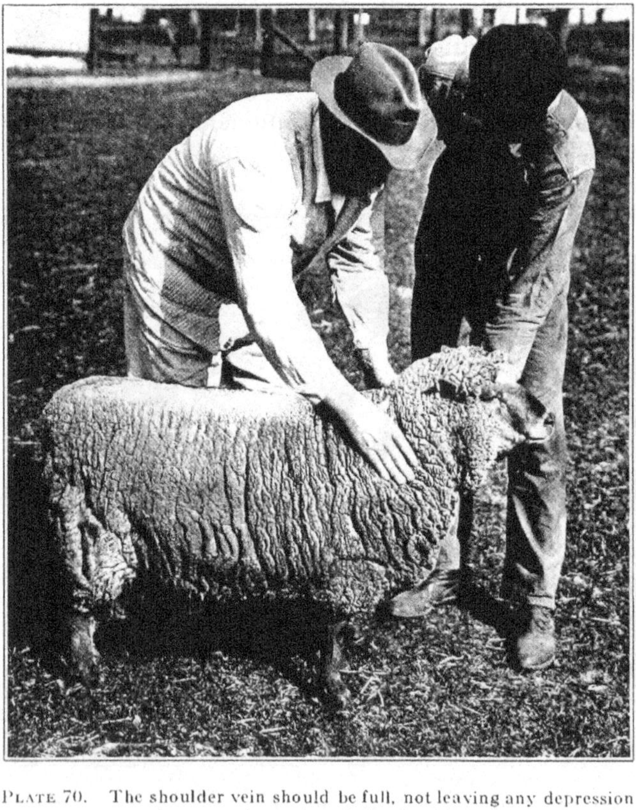

PLATE 70. The shoulder vein should be full, not leaving any depression between the neck and the shoulder.

THE SHOULDER VEIN.

The term shoulder vein does not mean that there is a particular vein at the place where the neck and shoulder join. It simply indicates the place where they meet. The shoulder vein of the sheep, corresponds to the place where the collar rests on the horse when in harness, and the neck should slope down from the head and join the shoulder in such a way that no depression is noticeable where they join, on top as well as on the sides. When so built, it adds to the value of the carcass, as butchers dislike the kind that are not well-developed in this part. It indicates a slim neck in front of it.

NOTING THE DEPTH OF CHEST.

By placing the right hand on top of the shoulder and the left hand between the fore legs, the depth of the chest may be estimated. A deep, broad chest is very essential in a sheep, rams as well as ewes. This part includes the shoulder, the breast, and the brisket. If the sheep is wide, broad, and deep in the chest, not only its greater weight and value of carcass is insured, but also its health. If the chest is narrow and shallow; the vital organs, the heart, and the lungs, which are at work there, are congested and cannot properly perform their functions, thereby causing a weak sheep that cannot

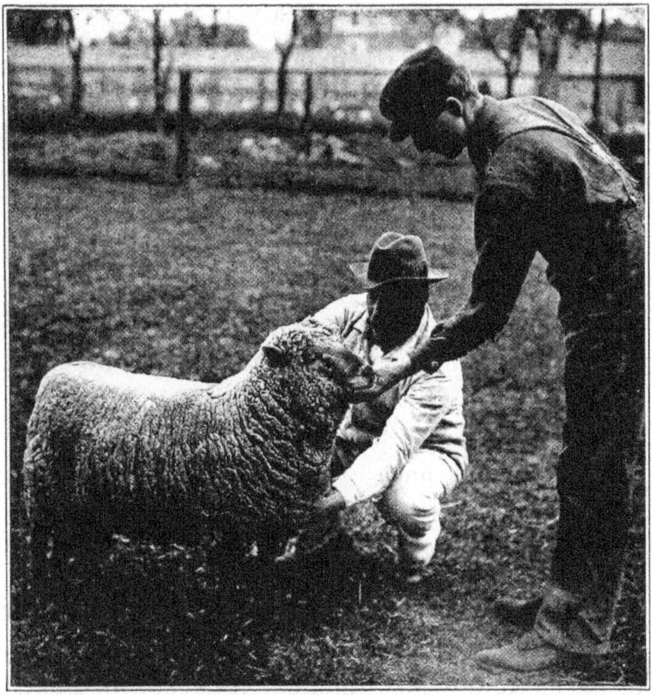

Plate 71. Estimating the depth of the chest by placing right hand on top of the shoulder, left hand between the fore legs.

withstand any attack of illness. On the other hand, the sheep that has a broad, deep chest, is strong, robust, healthy, and not nearly so susceptible to illness.

MEASURING THE WIDTH OF THE HEART GIRTH.

The width of the heart girth also aids in promoting the health of the sheep. If the sheep is broad and deep in the chest, but is light and narrow in the heart girth, the vital organs, some of which occupy space in it, are cramped too closely together. Furthermore, there would be a depression between the shoulder and the ribs which would destroy the square, symmetrical form of the sheep. A wide, deep, heart girth and chest insures a good constitution and is a very important factor.

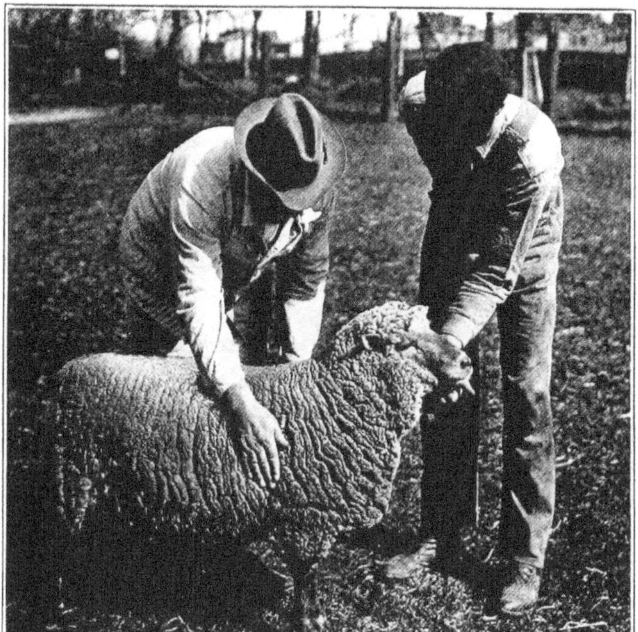

PLATE 72. Measuring the width of the heart girth. A large heart girth denotes a strong constitution.

COVERING, WIDTH, AND STRAIGHTNESS OF BACK.

The back includes the part of the sheep from the shoulders to the hips. From these parts the butcher gets the cuts of meat which sell for a higher

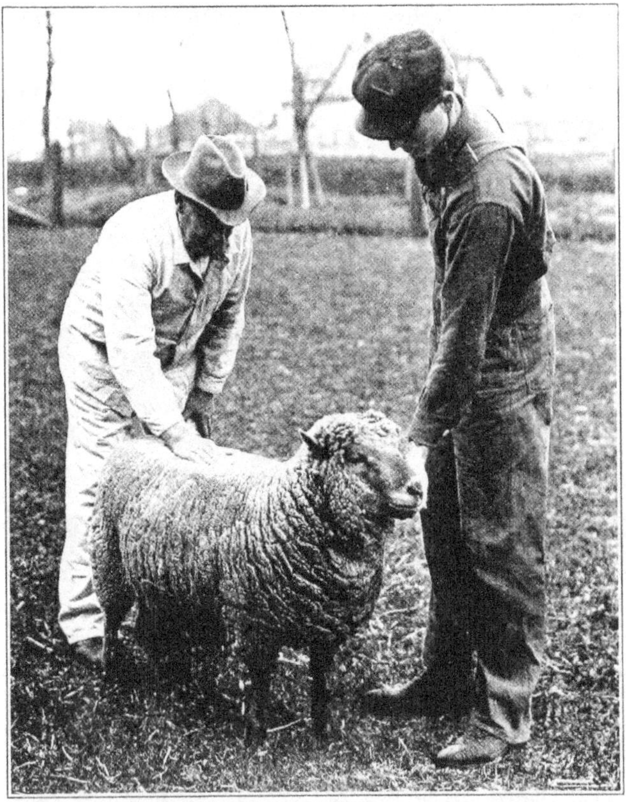

PLATE 73. Examining the straightness and covering of the back. This is a very essential part of a mutton sheep. The valuable cuts must be well-developed.

price at retail than any other part of the sheep. For this reason, the back first of all should be straight, with well-sprung ribs that give width to the back and good depth. Then the butcher can get many more pounds of these choice, higher-priced cuts and will be well repaid for the higher price he paid for the sheep with a broad back. The covering of flesh on the back is an important factor also. A broad, wide back with but little meat on it is not sought by the butcher, and since all mutton breeds go to the block eventually, a well-fleshed, straight, broad back is very desirable. The straightness of the back also adds to the good appearance of the sheep.

MEASURING THE WIDTH AND THICKNESS OF LOIN.

Measuring the width and thickness of the sheep's loin is another important point in rendering decisions, especially in judging fat sheep. For example, if two sheep are equally good in all other points, but one has a wider loin than the other, the latter should be given the preference, because from the loin the butcher gets many of the valuable cuts of meat. Usually when a sheep has a broad, fleshy, and well-developed back, it also has a broad, thick loin. In order that the smoothness of the fleece may not be marred and the sheep annoyed when the loin is being measured, the judge should place his hands straight on the loin, keep-

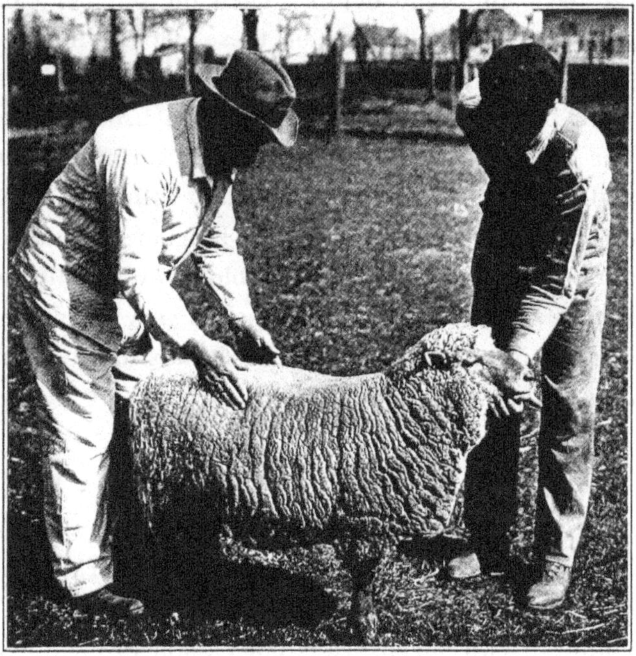

PLATE 74. The loin should be broad and thick. It is also one of the valuable cuts.

ing his fingers together as shown in the illustration.

NOTING THE WIDTH OF THE RUMP.

The idea of placing the two hands on the sheep's rump, is to find out whether the sheep carries its width out to the end of the body, straight and full. The reason for the importance of this examination is that the part back of the hips, called the rump

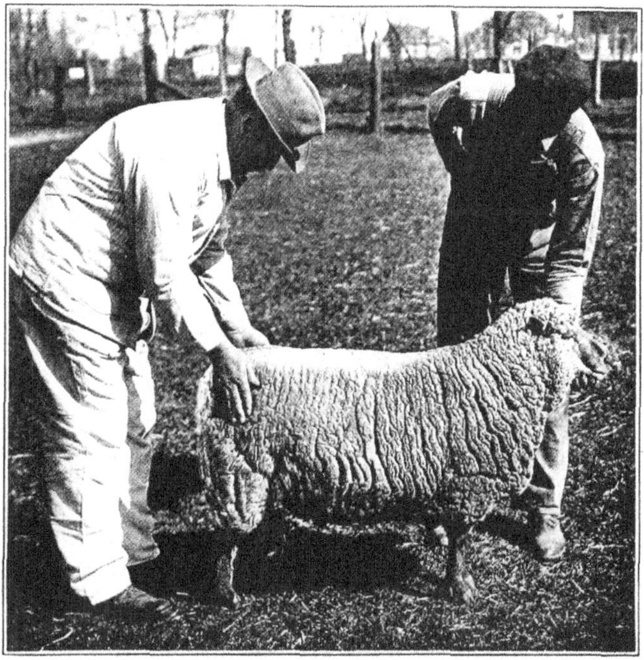

PLATE 75. Noting the width and fullness of rump. It is essential that the sheep carry its width to the end of the body.

or hindquarter, has the second highest priced meat. It is therefore essential that the sheep should be wide and full at this part of the body. Many sheep that are well-developed all over the body, often lack much in width of the rump. Instead of holding the straight line out to the end, they taper off to a sharp point. This defect is often not very noticeable, especially if the sheep has been trimmed. Much can be done by trimming to deceive the eye and to improve the looks of the sheep.

EXAMINING THE DEPTH OF TWIST.

By placing the left hand on top at the end of the rump, and the right hand between the two hind legs as shown in Figure 76, the judge can determine the fullness and depth of the sheep's twist. This portion when well-developed adds greatly to the value of the sheep, and consequently should receive the sharp attention of the judge. Sheep vary a great deal in this respect; some carry fullness of mutton down to the hocks, others nearly down, and still others are cut up between the legs like a goat. There is, of course, a natural difference in breeds with regard to this point, but it is desirable that each breed show a good development of the twist. The Southdown, perhaps, leads all other breeds in development here. It is well when judging rams to make sure at this time that they are fully developed and possess two testicles.

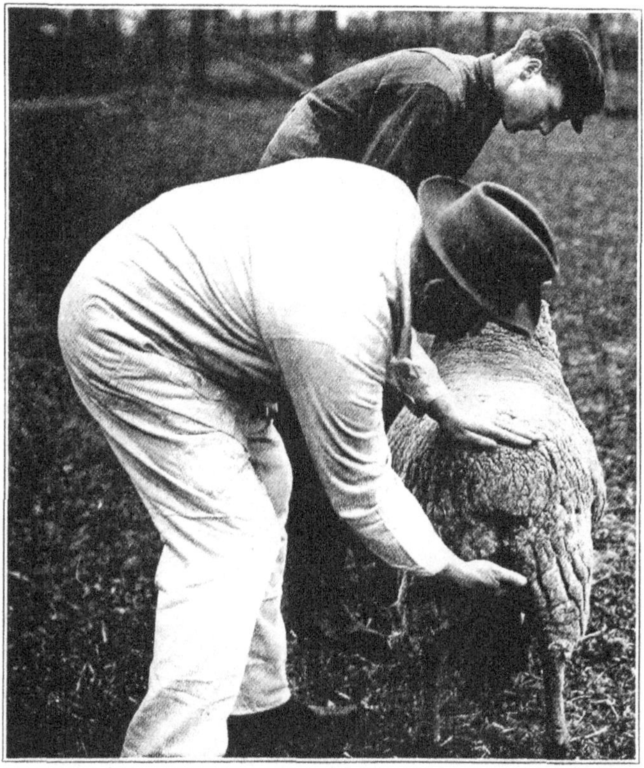

PLATE 76. A good sheep has a well-developed, full, deep twist to help make a big leg of mutton.

A LARGE LEG OF MUTTON DESIRABLE.

It is essential that each sheep should have a large, well-fleshed leg of mutton. Many, however, lack this highly desired development. A deep, full twist, and a well-fleshed thigh together furnish a

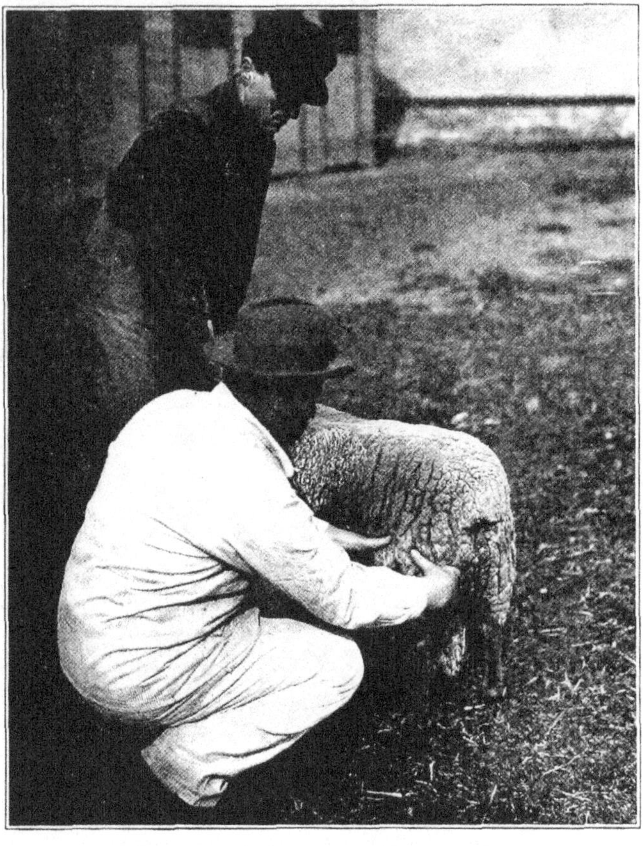

PLATE 77. Placing the left hand in front, the right at the rear of the leg, shows definitely the size of the leg of mutton.

large leg of mutton. Many people in this country, especially the wealthier classes, are great admirers of a good leg of mutton or lamb. Therefore, in selecting a ram to head the flock, particular attention should be paid to this point, since all good, as well as inferior qualities, are transmitted to the offspring by the sire and dam. By placing the two hands around the leg, as shown in Figure 77, the judge can quickly note the size and fleshiness of the leg.

EXAMINING THE FLEECE AND SKIN.

The proper method of parting the wool on the sheep's shoulder without marring the fleece is shown in Figure 78. When this is done correctly the fleece will part readily in layers. The length, fineness, lustre, crimp, and yolk is then noted. At the same time, the color of the skin should be taken into consideration. The skin should be of a pink color, indicating good health and good blood circulation. When a sheep is out of condition, caused by over-feeding, or perhaps, is infested with internal parasites, the color of the skin is rather pale. However, it should be remembered that some breeds of sheep naturally have a darker color of skin than others. The wool should be dense and of fine quality over the entire body.

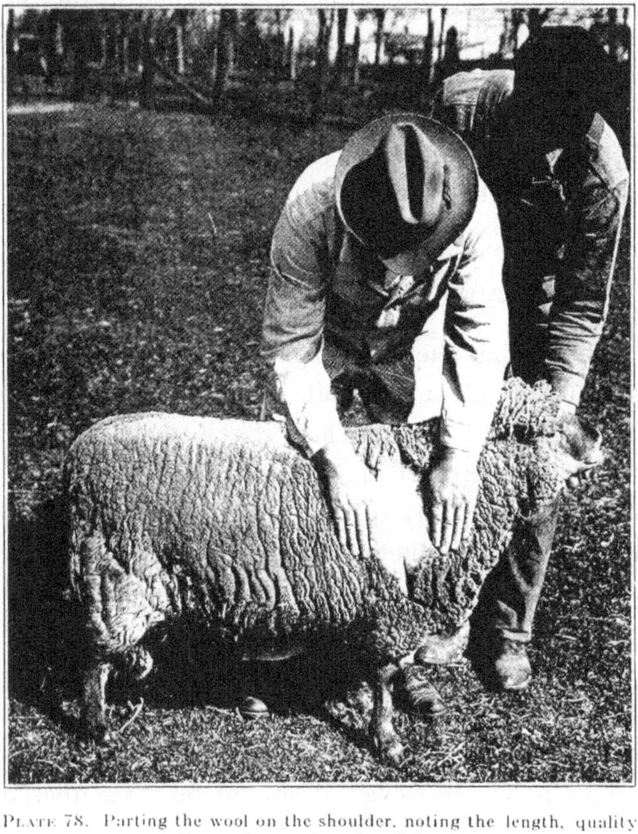

PLATE 78. Parting the wool on the shoulder, noting the length, quality of the wool, and the color of the skin.

NOTING THE QUALITY OF WOOL ON THE THIGH.

The best and finest wool on the sheep grows on the shoulder and heart girth, the poorest on the belly. It is difficult, however, to examine and com-

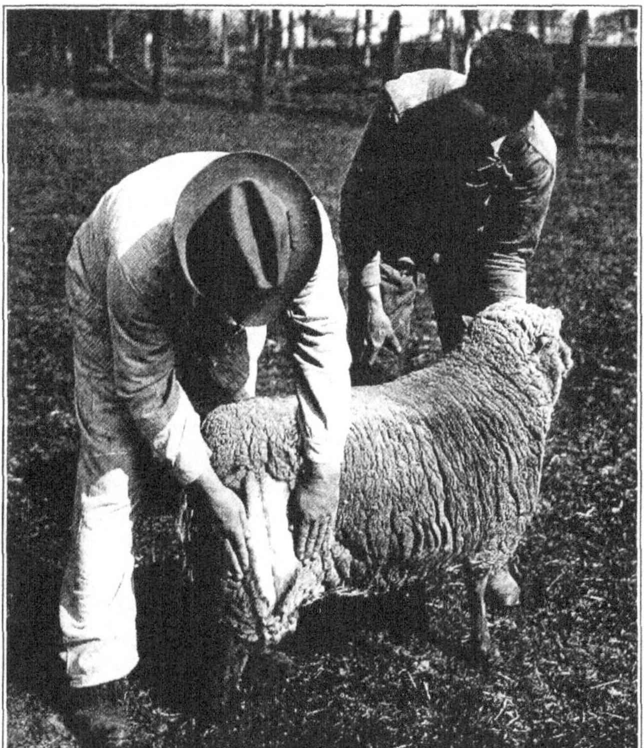

PLATE 79. Separate the wool on the thigh and compare it with that found on the shoulder. The quality in these parts should be as even as possible.

pare the wool on the under part of the body. The next poorest grows on the thigh. The evenness of quality is determined by these two parts. It should compare nearly uniformly in quality and fineness. It may be stated here that the writer in all his years of experience in raising and judging sheep has never found one sheep that was absolutely even in quality of the wool. Usually a slight difference can be noted, the wool on the thigh being a trifle coarser than that on the shoulder. It is very desirable to have the wool on both of these places as uniform in quality and fineness as possible. Figure 79 shows the proper place to make these comparisons.

CHAPTER XII.

CLASSIFICATION OF THE BREEDS OF SHEEP

Fewer breeds of sheep are raised on American farms than in Great Britain. Indeed, in England and Scotland, American flockowners would find not only the breeds common in this country, but also several which were practically unknown to them. Therefore, perhaps the best opportunity one could have to see all the various breeds without traveling over a large territory, would be to attend the great annual Royal show usually held in one of the larger cities in England. At this show, the breeds of sheep raised in England, Scotland, and Ireland are all assembled, making a grand display and leaving a deep impression on the person who is interested in seeing so many different kinds on exhibition. This show offers an excellent chance to study and compare the different breeds.

At the present time, only about twelve breeds are familiar to American shepherds. These twelve recognized breeds are divided into three distinct groups, namely, medium or middle wools, long or coarse wools, and fine wools.

The medium or middle wools consist of eight different breeds, as follows: Shropshire Down,

Oxford Down, Hampshire Down, Southdown, Dorset Horn, Cheviot, Suffolk, and Tunis. The last two mentioned are not very numerous in the United States.

The long or coarse wools consist of the following: Cotswold, Lincoln, Leicester, and Romney Marsh or Kent. There are not yet many of the last named in America.

The fine wools consist of the following breeds: American also called Spanish Merino, Delaine Merino, and the Rambouillet or French Merino.

The writer has been asked many times which is the best breed to raise. The beginner should determine this matter himself by considering the breed he likes best, and the one which is best adapted to the kind of land upon which he wishes to raise sheep. If his land is hilly and rough, the smaller breeds will do better than the larger ones,. as it will be easier for them to climb around the hills. The larger breeds are better suited for the more level areas.

Sheep are no longer raised merely for their wool. Now mutton is considered first, and wool is looked upon as a by-product. A breed of sheep that has a good mutton form and at the same time shears a fleece of good market quality, seems to be in favor among flockmasters, and no doubt is the most profitable.

Climatic conditions must also be considered in determining the kind of breed to raise. If the farmer intends to raise lambs for an early market, the warmer states are more favorable than others. It may be said that each breed will thrive and do well if the climate corresponds as nearly as possible to that of the country from which the breed originates. The beginner should make a careful study of the conditions in his locality, and select the breed best suited to his taste and conditions.

THE SHROPSHIRE.

The Shropshire is the most popular breed in America at the present time. This may be accounted for by the fact that it is a sheep of beautiful style and appearance, with a good mutton form, and has a fine fleece of good weight and market quality. In size it ranks between the Southdown and the other middle wool breeds.

The best Shropshire is wooled from nose to toes. Its face and legs are a rich dark brown color. The head is short and broad between the ears, with full prominent eyes. The ears are small, carried well erect, and covered preferably with fine curls of wool on top. The neck is short, shoulders smooth, and the chest very deep, with the brisket projecting well forward. The back is straight and broad with a good spring of ribs. The hindquar-

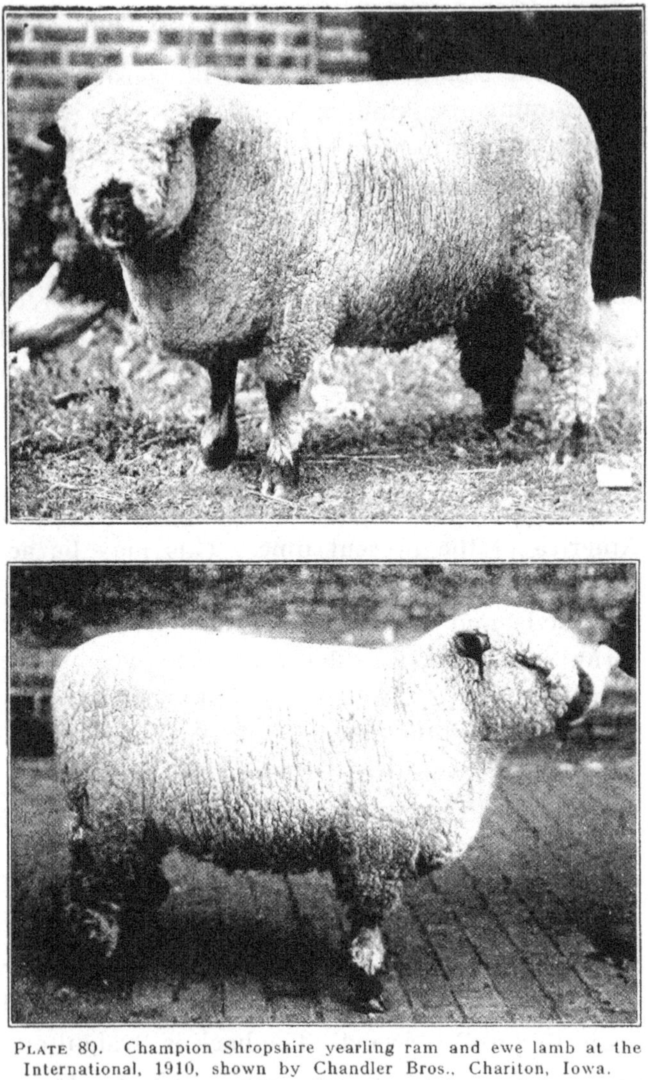

PLATE 80. Champion Shropshire yearling ram and ewe lamb at the International, 1910, shown by Chandler Bros., Chariton, Iowa. Both show very good Shropshire type and characteristics.

ters are full and deep with a well-developed leg of mutton. The legs are short and straight, of good sized bone, and set squarely under the body. The skin is of light cherry color and free from dark spots. The fleece when full grown is generally about three inches long and contains considerable yolk. There should be no horns or stubs on a purebred Shropshire, nor should there be any but white wool on its whole body and head.

POINTS OF EXCELLENCE FOR SHROPSHIRE SHEEP.

(1)—TYPE AND GENERAL APPEARANCE.

An alert, attractive, and stylish appearance, showing at a glance the true characteristics of the Shropshire 30

(2)—FORM AND CONSTITUTION

Head.—To impress at once the Shropshire characteristics.

Heads of Rams.—To be masculine as indicated by a broad nostril, short, broad between ears and eyes.

Neck.—Short and muscular fitting into shoulders in graceful outlines.

Heads of Ewes.—To be feminine in appearance, medium in length, but not delicate.

Neck.—Not so strong as in the ram. In all cases head and face nicely covered with wool; ears, short and erect; eyes, bright; color of face, brown to a clear dark (not sooty black).

Body.—Well proportioned with shoulders so placed as to fit in evenly to a deep wide brisket. A full heart-girth; broad level back; ribs well sprung with straight underline; loins thick-fleshed; fore and hind flank deep; a low coupled twist, and full leg of mutton.

Legs.—Brown to clear dark color (not sooty black), well set apart, short and straight with strong upright pasterns.

Size.—When fully matured and in proper breeding condition,

Rams should weigh not less than 175 to 250 pounds and Ewes not less than 140 to 180 pounds 35

(3)—FLESHING

While the body should be well formed with the full outline pleasing to the eye, yet it is the quality and quantity of flesh not fat, which gives value to the carcass. Therefore the parts furnishing the high-priced cuts should be fully developed.

The back, loins and legs, should be so fleshed as to show a large percentage of flesh compared with the other parts of the body, at the same time symmetry must prevail throughout.

Strong bone in legs conformable with size of body usually goes with a large proportion of lean meat to fat in the finished carcass. . 25

(4)—FLEECE AND SKIN.

Fleece of good length, elastic to the touch, medium fine and slightly crimped, free from black fibre and hairiness. Ram's scrotum to be well covered with wool.

Rams should shear 8 to 15 pounds of wool and ewes 7 to 11

Skin to be a bright cherry or clear color and comparatively free from dark spots. 10

OBJECTIONS.

Long narrow head with long ears and neck; long legs; black wool on head to any noticeable extent; failure of wool to meet closely at the junction of facewool and on cheeks; white spots on face and legs; crooked spine; light flanks, with long weak pasterns; spotted skin; narrow chest showing lack of constitution.

DISQUALIFICATION FOR REGISTRY.

Such lack of type as to render it doubtful to a breeder what the breed is; **Horns** or **Stubs, not Scurs.** Heads quite bare of wool.

THE OXFORD.

The Oxford originated from a cross between the Cotswold and the Hampshire. As a result of the combination of the blood from these two large breeds, the Oxford today is a big sheep, and the length of its wool adds further to its large appearance. A true type Oxford shows an abundance of style and carriage.

It is a large-framed, heavy-boned sheep. The color of the face and legs varies considerably, some being brown and others of a much darker color. The same variation is evident with regard to the amount of wool on the face and cheeks, some having more wool on these parts than others. The typical Oxford, however, has a heavy bunch of wool standing out prominently on the forehead between the eyes. Many have a little white spot on the end of the nose. The head is large but not coarse; broad over the poll with a much larger ear than the Shropshire. The body is well proportioned and carries out its width particularly well at the rear. The wool is long and somewhat coarse, and is often lacking in density. Some, however, possess a shorter, finer, and denser fleece than others. The size of this sheep and its heavy shearing quality have made it popular in America. Oxford rams have been extensively and successfully used for crossing on ordinary native and western ewes to improve the size and wool production.

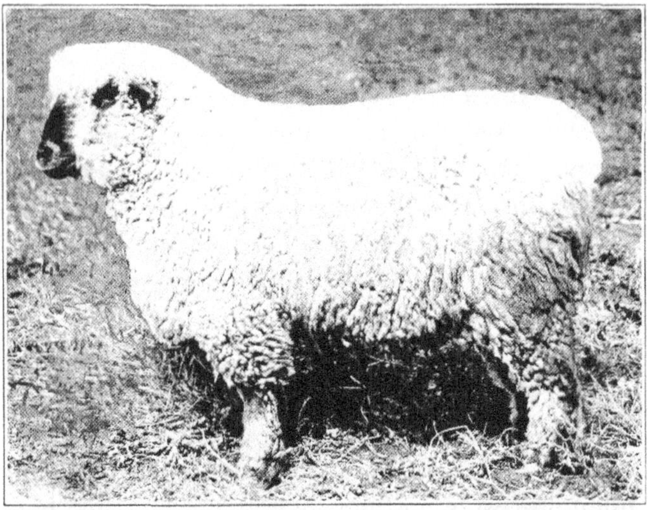

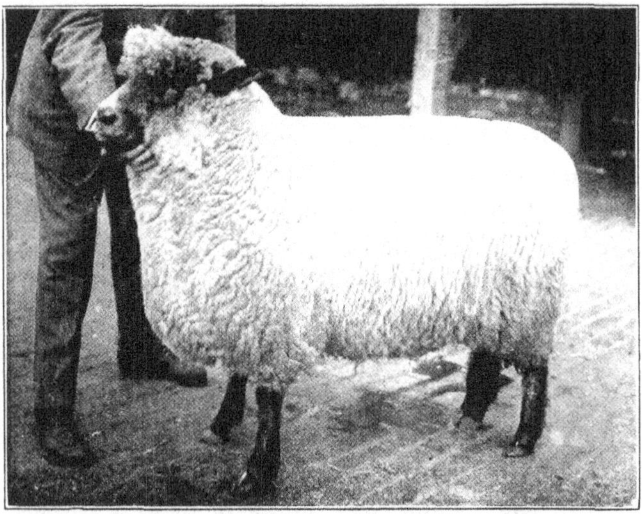

PLATE 81. A good, typical pair of Oxfords. Champion Oxford ram winner of many prizes. Champion Oxford ewe at the International, 1910. Both sheep shown by George McKerrow, Pewaukee, Wis.

SCALE OF POINTS FOR OXFORD DOWN SHEEP.

IN FOUR DIVISIONS.

Breed type	30
Constitution	25
Mutton form and quality	30
Wool	15

SUB-DIVISIONS.

BREED TYPE FOR ANIMALS.

Form of a good general appearance, made by a well balanced conformation, free from coarseness in any part, and showing good style both at rest and in motion	15
Head of moderate length and width between the ears and between the eyes, and well covered with wool over poll and down to the eyes. Color of face an even dark gray or brown, either with or without gray spot on tip of nose	6
When fully matured and in good condition Rams should weigh 250 to 350 lbs., Ewes, 180 to 275 lbs.	5
Ears medium size, not too thick and of an even brown or dark gray color	2
Legs short, strong in bone, flat and of even dark gray or brown color, placed squarely under the body and well apart	2

CONSTITUTION.

Large around the heart and wide and full in the chest	10
The movement must be bold and vigorous	5
Eyes bold, prominent and bright	4
Skin bright pink in color	3
Neck strong and muscular in rams and well set on in both sexes	3

MUTTON FORM AND QUALITY.

Wide and straight on top of shoulders, back, loin and rump, from base of neck to tail	15
Full shoulders and thighs, well meated both inside and outside	5
Flanks well filled and strong so as to make the lower lines of the body as straight as possible, and side lines straight or rather full	4
The whole carcass evenly covered with good, well marbled meat	6

WOOL.

Fleece of moderate length, close and of even quality, covering the whole carcass, well and free from black patches upon the body, neck or head	15
Total	100

THE HAMPSHIRE.

Twelve or fifteen years ago this breed was not found in very great numbers, but in late years it has become quite popular in this country, especially in the western states. It is a large sheep about the equal in weight of the Oxford. The lambs mature early, since they are large at birth, and are forced ahead by the remarkable milk flow of their mothers. Hence their owner is enabled to get lambs of the desirable weight and flesh on the market at the age of from seventy-five to ninety days, when they command a high price. The writer has seen lambs of this breed that weighed twenty-four and twenty-six pounds when fifteen days old. The Hampshire is also a very prolific sheep.

The color of the head and legs is preferably a rich black. The head is somewhat long and the ears a little drooped. The frame of the body is long and straight and is covered with short dense wool, having but little yolk. The wool on the head usually extends a little beyond the eyes and cheeks, forming, as it is called, a "cap." Little wool is found on the front legs below the knees, the hind legs are slightly wooled below the hocks. This breed, like the Oxford, is used to a great extent for crossbreeding in the western states.

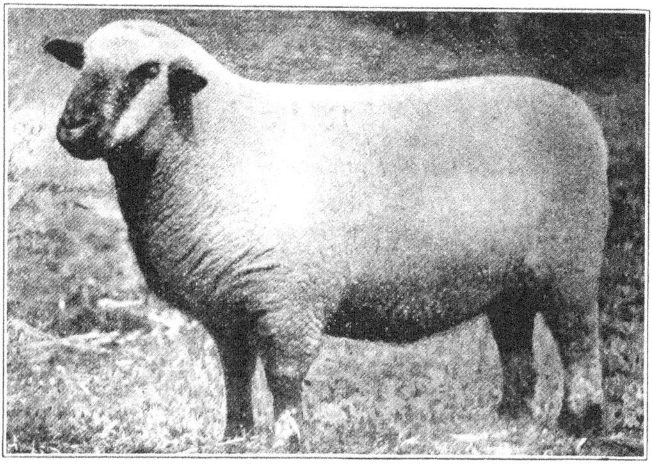

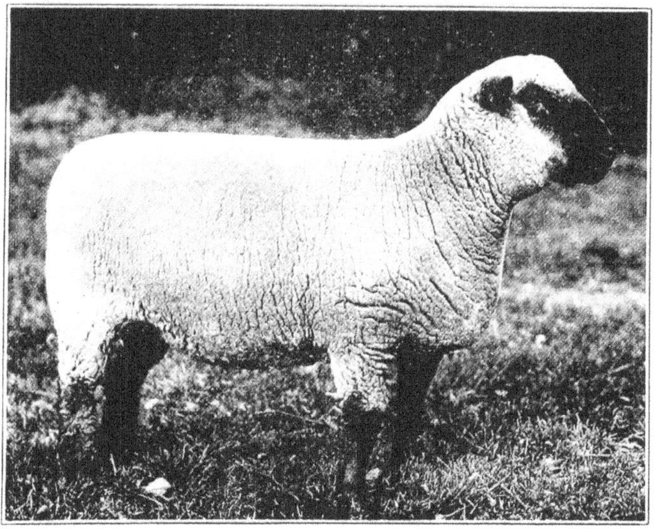

PLATE 82. The Donerail, Kentucky, Walnut Hall Stud ram, "Britain" who was never defeated in England or in America. A prize winning Hampshire yearling ewe in England and America. Courtesy F. Babbage, London, England.

STANDARD OF EXCELLENCE FOR HAMPSHIRE SHEEP

HEAD AND LEGS.

Head—Moderately large, but not coarse; well covered with wool on forehead and cheeks.

Nostrils—Wide.

Color (head and legs)—Dark brown or black.

Eyes—Prominent and lustrous.

Ears—Moderately long and thin, and dark brown or black color.

Legs—Well under outside of body, straight, with good size of bone, black.

NECK, SHOULDERS AND CHEST.

Neck—A regular taper from shoulders to head, without any hollow in front of shoulders, set high up on body.

Shoulders—Sloping, full, and not higher than the line of back and neck.

Chest—Deep and full in the heart place, with breast prominent and full.

BODY.

Back—Straight, with full spring of rib.

Loin—Wide and straight, without depression in front of hips.

Quarters—Long from hips to rump, without sloping, and deep in thigh. Broad in hips and rump, with full hams. Inside of thigh full.

SCALE OF POINTS.

Head—Size and shape, 5; ears and eyes, 3; color, 5; legs and feet, 2	15
Neck, shoulders and breast—Neck, 5; shoulders, 10; chest and breast, 15	30
Body—Back and loins, 15; ribs, 5	20
Quarters—Length, 10; width, 10; twist, 5	25
Wool—Forehead and cheeks, 2; belly, well covered, 3; quality, 5	10
Total	100

THE SOUTHDOWN.

This little aristocratic breed is one of the oldest in history. It is generally called the "gentleman's sheep." The form of the Southdown meets more nearly with the ideal market requirements than any other breed. This breed is not as popular as it should be. In the southern and eastern states, it is appreciated more than in the middle and western states. The chief reason for their unpopularity is probably the fact that they do not grow as large as other breeds and do not shear as heavy fleeces.

The Southdown, with its excellent mutton form and qualities, is built low to the ground and has a very compact, symmetrical form. The hindquarters are very full and deep, carrying meat far down to the hocks. The head and ears are short, but attractive. The face and legs should be of a uniform gray, or mouse color. The neat body is wrapped in a rather short, but extremely dense fleece, with but little yolk in it. Although the fleece is rather light in weight, they produce the finest quality of wool, next to the Merino families. Their small appearance often deceives one as to their real weight.

Among the many breeds the Southdown, from the writer's observation, is the most economical feeder, as it keeps up the longest in flesh when the

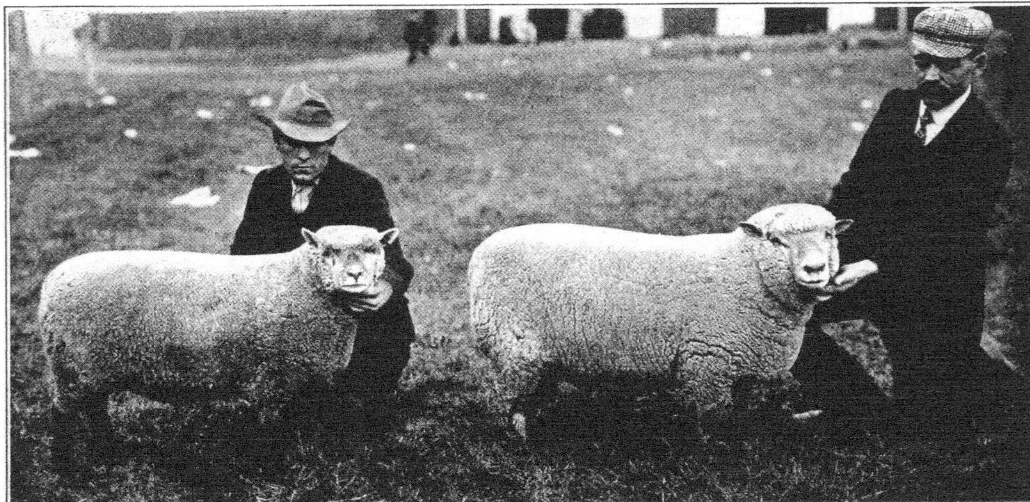

PLATE 83. An undefeated Southdown ram and ewe. Both have won first prize and champion wherever shown at state fairs and larger shows. Shown by George Allen, Ontario, Canada.

feed becomes scarce. It is often said that there is more mutton on a square inch of Southdown than on any other breed, a fact difficult to dispute. On the block, the Southdown is hard to beat, for when dressed, it shows a beautiful marbling or mixture of fat and lean meat.

STANDARD OF EXCELLENCE FOR SOUTHDOWN SHEEP.

Head medium in size and hornless, fine, carried well up, the forehead or face well covered with wool, especially between the ears and on the cheeks, and in ewe slightly dished	5
Lips and under jaw fine and thin	1
Ears rather small, tolerably wide apart, covered with fine hair, and carried with a lively back and forth movement	2
Eyes full and bright	3
Face a uniform tint of brown, or gray, or mouse color	3
Neck short, fine at the head, but nicely tapering, and broad and straight on top at the shoulders	4
Shoulders broad and full, smoothly joining the neck with the back	5
Breast wide, deep and projecting well forward, the forelegs standing wide apart	5
Back and loin broad and straight from shoulders to rump	7
Ribs well arched extending far backward, the last projecting more than the others	6
Rump broad, square and full, with tail well set up	6
Hips wide, with little space between them and last ribs	6
Thighs full and well let down in twist, the legs standing well apart	6
Limbs short and fine in bone, and in color to agree with the face	3
Forelegs well wooled and carrying mutton to the knees, but free from meat below	2
Hind legs well filled with mutton and wooled to the hocks, neat and clean below	2
Belly straight and covered with wool, the flank extending so as to form a line parallel with the back or top line	5
Fleece compact, the whole body well covered with moderately long and close wool white in color, carrying some yolk	12
Form throughout smooth and symmetrical, with no coarseness in any part	9
General appearance spirited and attractive, with a determined look, a proud and firm step, indicating constitutional vigor and thorough breeding	8
Total	100

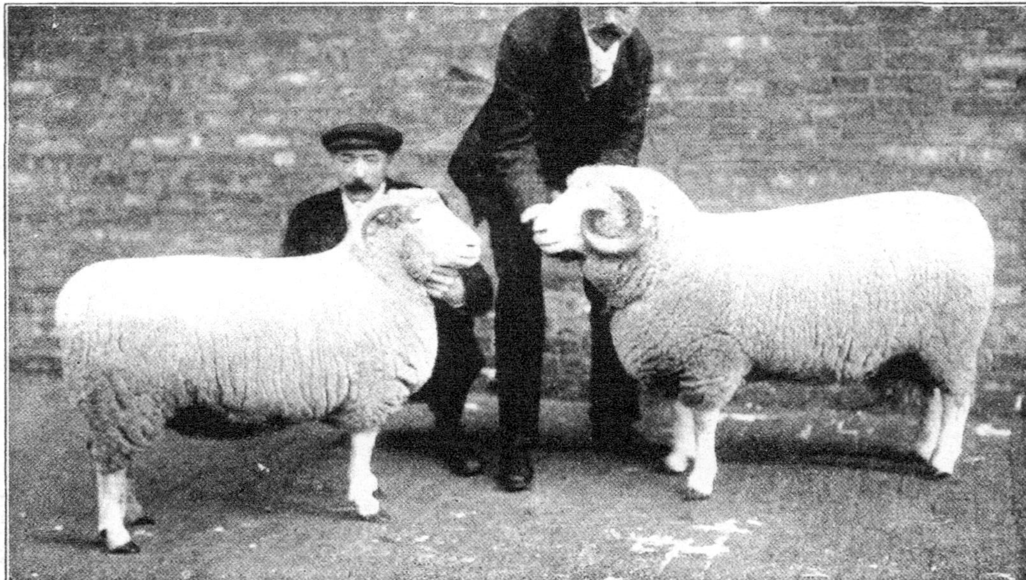

PLATE 84. First prize Dorset ram and ewe lamb at the International, 1910; shown by Heart's Delight Farm, Chazey, New York.

THE DORSET HORN.

This breed is one of the medium wools originating in Dorsetshire, England, and is used to a great extent in the production of winter, or so-called "hot-house" lambs which are marketed generally between Christmas and Easter or even later. In the writer's experience, there is no other breed more profitable for early lamb production, where there is a good market for them. The Dorset can be bred almost any time in the year and if desired often produces two crops of lambs in one year. It is very prolific and is an extremely heavy, rich milker. It is a rather large, round-bodied sheep with strong legs and bone. Both sexes have horns, those of the ram being larger and more twisted than those of the ewe.

The color of the head, face, and legs is white. No black or other color should be found on it, not even on the hoofs. It is fairly short in the legs, and the body is of great length. The fleece is of fine quality, of medium length, very white in color, and has little yolk. The skin is, perhaps, of a pinker color than can be found on any other breed of sheep.

SCALE OF POINTS FOR DORSET HORN SHEEP.

Head.—Neat, face white, nostrils large, well covered on crown and under jaws with wool	5
Horns.—Small and gracefully curving forward rather close to jaw	5
Eyes.—Prominent and bright	2
Ears.—Medium size covered with short white hair	2
Neck.—Short, symmetrical, strongly set on shoulders, gradually tapering to junction of head	5
Shoulders.—Broad and full, joining neck forward and chine backward with no depression at either point. (important)	15
Brisket.—Wide and full, forward, chest full and deep	8
Fore Flank.—Quite full, showing little depression behind shoulder	8
Back and loin.—Wide and straight, from which ribs should spring with a fine, circular arch	10
Quarters.—Wide and full, with mutton extending down to hocks	10
Belly.—Straight on under line	3
Fleece.—Medium grade, of even quality presenting a smooth surface and extending over belly and well down on legs	12
General conformation.—Of the mutton type, body moderately long; short, stout legs, placed squarely under body, skin pink, appearance attractive	15
Total	100

THE CHEVIOT.

The Cheviot breed of sheep has been well-known in Scotland for more than two hundred years. It is considered in that country as a mountain sheep,

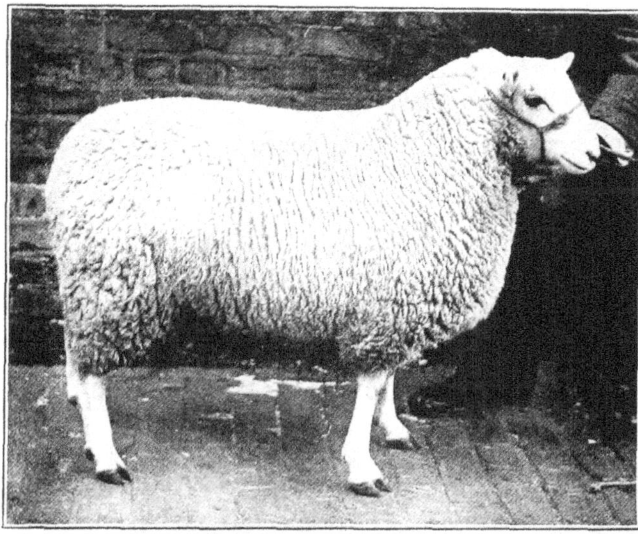

PLATE 85. Cheviot ram lamb winning first prize at the International 1910; shown by F. L. Postle and Son, Ohio.

for no hill seems too high for it to climb. It is very hardy, alert and active. Its appearance and movement are very attractive. It is best suited for rough, hilly land, which cannot be utilized for other farm animals. In the writer's observation, it thrives far better on hilly land than on the lower bottom land.

This breed is characterized by its blocky form, and by a fairly dense wool of good length. As a rule, it is somewhat sharp over the shoulders, but has a broad back, with good full hindquarters. The head is short with a clean-cut, white face. The

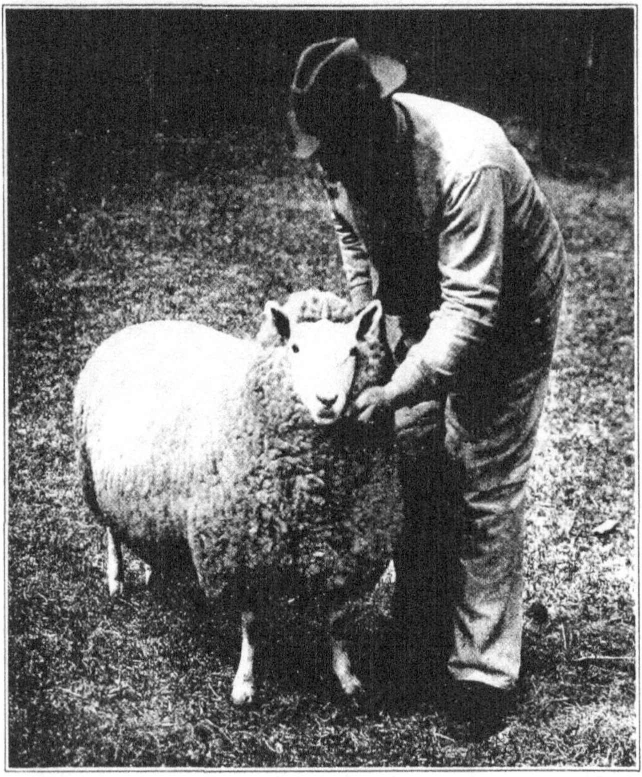

PLATE 86. A very typical Cheviot ewe owned by the University of Wisconsin.

nose is black and the eye prominent. Black spots, which are not objectionable, are often found on the ears. The ears are carried more erect than those of any other breed. The legs are fine-boned. The front legs are round, the hind legs are flat. The hoofs are black. The wool grows up close to the ears, forming a high crest, but from there on forward to the head and face no wool, only hair, should be seen. There should be no mixture of red hairs on the head, ears, or legs of the Cheviot. The rams are allowed to have horns not exceeding one inch in length.

STANDARD AND SCALE OF POINTS FOR JUDGING CHEVIOT SHEEP.

General conformation and quality—Deep and full breast and large through chest. Back: wide and straight with well sprung. deep ribs, legs well placed and leg of mutton full and thick. Body well fleshed, skin pink with no blue or dark coloring, fleece compact and medium fine, bone strong and fine, general appearance graceful, symmetrical, active	20
Size—In good flesh when fully matured a twenty-four months' old ram should weigh not less than 225 lbs., and a ewe not less than 150 lbs.	10
Head—Should be medium short and broad with ample breadth between the eyes. Ears should be of medium length and usually erect when at repose. Head covered with clear white hairs, extending from nostrils to back of poll. Ridge of head from between eyes to nostrils straight or slightly arched with females and more strongly arched or Roman with rams. Color of tip of nose black	15
Body—Well proportioned, having notable depth, with thickness on top and at flanks. Loins should be very broad and thick, shoulders should set well back and be smoothly covered, and crops be full and well arched. The rump should be long, broad and level	20
Legs—Should be short, well set apart and be covered with clean white hair with no wool below hocks and knees. The hind legs should be flat and deep below hocks. Pasterns should be strong and not show weakness, supporting the body well.	10
Feet—Symmetrical, squarely placed when in repose and hoofs black in color	5
Fleece—Should cover the body completely to behind the poll and ears and down to knees and hocks. Under part of the body should be well covered. In mature animals should be not less than three inches long for annual growth and be compact and of medium wool class. Rams should shear at least 12 pounds and ewes 8 when in mature form to be desirable representatives of the breed	20

OBJECTIONS.

Scurs on the head, black spots on the head, flesh colored or spotted skin about the nostrils, hair about the thighs or kemp on the body, reddish or sandy hair on head or legs, lack of wool on under part of body.

Disqualifications—All male lambs shall be ineligible to registration, if having scurs or horns exceeding one inch in length.

THE SUFFOLK.

This breed belongs to the middle wools. It is a large-framed sheep with rather long legs. The body is round in form, and very lengthy. The head is large, the face very black, and the ears long and

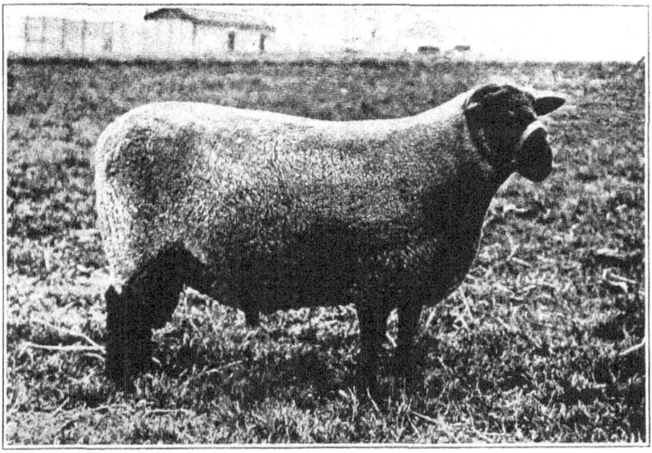

PLATE 87. Champion Suffolk ram at English shows. Courtesy of Suffolk Sheep Society, E. M. Prentice, Secretary; Ipswich, England

black. The fine-boned, black legs are bare of wool below the knees and hocks. The wool is short, but dense. The head from the ears forward is entirely bare of wool like that of the Cheviot. The skin is pink in color and the wool is a little grayish white. The Suffolk is known as a very hardy breed, although it is not very popular in this country. In Canada there are a number of flocks of this breed. At the English fat stock shows, Suffolk fat lambs in competition with many other breeds have often won the grand championship prize.

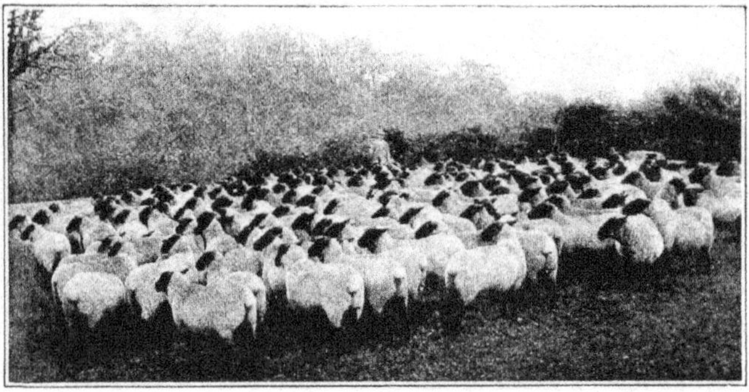

PLATE 88. Champion flock of Suffolk ewes. Courtesy of Suffolk Sheep Society, E. M. Prentice, Secretary; Ipswich, England.

SCALE OF POINTS FOR SUFFOLK SHEEP.

Head.—Hornless: Face black and long, and muzzle moderately fine—especially in ewes. (A small quantity of clean white wool on the forehead not objected to). Ears, a medium length, black and fine texture. Eyes, bright and full	25
Neck.—Moderate length and well set (In rams stronger, with a good crest)	5
Shoulder.—Broad and oblique	5
Chest.—Deep and wide	5
Back and loin—Long, level, and well covered with meat and muscle; Tail broad and well set up. The ribs long and well sprung, with a full flank	20
Legs and feet.—Straight and black, with fine and flat bone. Woolled to knees and hocks, clean below. Fore legs set well apart. Hind legs well filled with mutton	20
Belly (also scrotum of rams.)—Well covered with wool	5
Fleece.—Moderately short; close fine fibre without tendency to mat or felt together, and well defined, *i.e.*, not shading off into dark wool or hair	10
Skin.—Fine, soft, and pink color	5
Total	100

THE TUNIS.

This is a breed not yet very well known in this country, its native home being northern Africa. It is often called the fat tailed sheep. The breed

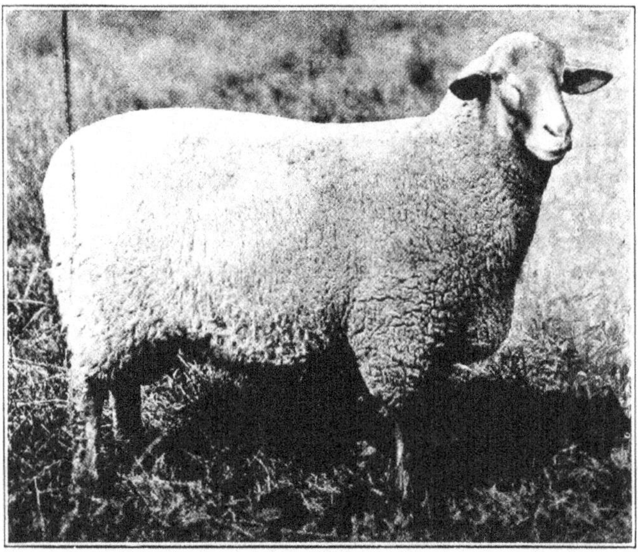

PLATE 89. Champion Tunis ram, Ohio State Fair, 1915. Property of Frank Hartman, Indiana.

is claimed to be an early lamb producer, similar to the Dorset. The Tunis is of medium size, has a fairly long fleece, either white, brown, or even grayish in color. On the long and rather narrow head, there is not much wool. The ears are heavy and long and droop forward. The color of the face and legs is often a speckled brown or white. The legs are small in bone and in most cases free from wool below the knees and hocks. Up to this time, but few men have engaged in raising this breed.

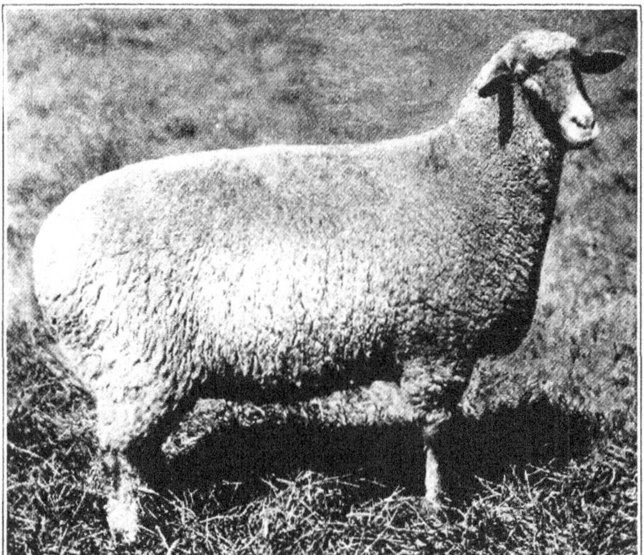

PLATE 90. Champion Tunis ewe, shown by Raymond Hays, Indiana.

SCALE OF POINTS FOR TUNIS SHEEP.

Blood.—Imported from Tunis or a perfect line of ancestors extending back to the flock owned and bred by Judge Richard Peters, of Pennsylvania	20
Constitution.—Healthful countenance, lively look, head erect, deep chest, ribs well arched, round body with good length; strong, straight back, muscles fine and firm	15
Fleece.—Medium length, medium quality, medium quantity; color white, sometimes tinctured with gray; evenness throughout	10
Covering.—Body and neck well covered with wool; legs bare, or slightly covered; face free of wool and covered with fine hair	10
Form.—Body straight, broad and well proportioned; small bone; breast wide and prominent in front; tail should be docked short	12
Head.—Small and hornless, or nearly so, tapering to end of nose; face and nose clean, in color, brown and white; ears broad, pendulous, and covered with fine hair, in color, brown to white	10
Neck.—Medium in length, well placed on shoulders, small and tapering	5
Legs.—Short; color brown and white, wooled below the knee not objectionable	6
Size.—In fair condition when fully matured rams should weigh 150 pounds and upward; ewes, 120 pounds and upward	6
General Appearance.—Good carriage; head well up; quick, elastic movements, showing symmetry of form and uniformity of character throughout	6
Total	100

THE COTSWOLD.

A typical Cotswold is a big-framed, tall sheep, stylish in appearance. The color of the face, ears, and legs is white or white mixed with some brown. The wool extends over the poll of the head, and hangs in ringlets or locks of varying lengths down over the face, covering it almost entirely. All over the body the wool hangs in long wavy curls, a characteristic of this breed not found as much in the other long wools. The wool on the hindquarters is often somewhat hairy. However, the fleece as a whole is nice and bright, and since it does not contain a great deal of yolk, there is not much shrinkage when it is washed, and it therefore sells well. As a rule, the Cotswold has a very straight back of good handling quality. Strong bone and masculinity characterize this breed.

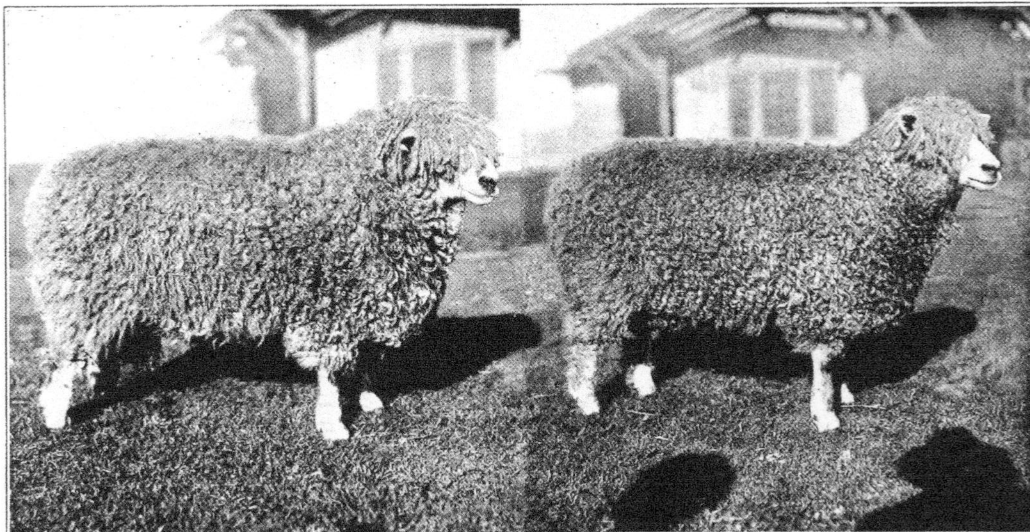

PLATE 91. Grand champion yearling Cotswold ram and ewe at the Panama Pacific Exposition, 1915. Bred and owned by F. A. Koser, Rickreall, Oregon. Ram weighed 360 pounds, ewe 253 pounds.

STANDARD OF EXCELLENCE AND SCALE OF POINTS FOR COTSWOLD RAM.

Ram—Head not too fine, moderately small and broad between the eyes and nostrils, but without a short, thick appearance, and in young animals well covered on the crown with long, lustrous wool	8
Face either white or slightly mixed with gray, or white dappled with brown	4
Nostrils wide and expanded; nose dark	1
Eyes prominent but mild looking	2
Ears broad, long, moderately thin and covered with short hair .	4
Collar full from breast and shoulders, tapering gradually all the way to where the neck and head join. The neck should be short, thick and strong, indicating constitutional vigor, and free from coarse and loose skin	6
Shoulders broad and full, and at the same time join so gradually to the collar forward and chine backward as not to leave the least hollow in either place	8
Fore legs—The mutton on the arm or fore thigh should come quite to the knee. Leg upright with heavy bone, being clear from superfluous skin, with wool to fetlock, and may be mixed with gray	4
Breast broad and well forward, keeping the legs wide apart; girth or chest, full and deep	10
Fore flank quite full, not showing hollow behind the shoulders .	5
Back and loin broad, flat and straight, from which the ribs must spring with a fine circular arch	12
Belly straight on underline	3
Quarters long and full, with mutton quite down to the hock -	8
Hock should stand neither in nor out	2
Twist or junction inside the thighs, deep, wide and full, which, with a broad breast, will keep the legs open and upright . .	5
Fleece—The whole body should be covered with long lustrous wool	18
Total	100

STANDARD OF EXCELLENCE AND SCALE OF POINTS FOR COTSWOLD EWE.

Ewe—Head moderately fine, broad between the eyes and nostrils, but without a short, thick appearance, and well covered on crown with long, lustrous wool	8
Face either white or slightly mixed with gray, or white dappled with brown	4
Nostrils wide and expanded; nose dark	1
Eyes prominent but mild looking	2
Ears broad, long, moderately thin, and covered with short hair .	4
Collar full from breast and shoulders, tapering gradually all the way to where the neck and head join; the neck should be fine and graceful, and free from coarse and loose skin	5
Shoulders broad and full, and at the same time join so gradually to the collar forward and chine backward as not to leave the least hollow in either place	8
Fore legs—The mutton on the arm or fore thigh should come quite to the knee; leg upright with heavy bone, being clear from superfluous skin, with wool to fetlock, and may be mixed with gray .	4
Breast broad and well forward, keeping the legs wide apart; girth or chest, full and deep	10
Fore flank quite full, not showing hollow behind the shoulder . .	4
Back and loin broad, flat and straight, from which the ribs must spring with a fine circular arch	12
Belly straight on underline	5
Quarters long and full, with mutton quite down to the hock . .	8
Hock should stand neither in nor out	2
Twist or junction inside the thighs, deep, wide and full, which, with a broad breast, will keep the legs open and upright	5
Fleece—The whole body should be covered with long, lustrous wool	18
Total	100

THE LINCOLN.

The Lincoln is shorter and more compactly built than the Cotswold. The face and legs are white with an occasional bluish tinge. The back is very strong and thickly fleshed. The wool is much longer than that of the Cotswold. It usually parts on the middle of the back and when full grown hangs down on each side in long broad locks. The wool is coarser than that of some of the other long wool breeds and has small curls at the ends. Often this breed has locks of wool hanging down over the face, but these are much shorter than those of the Cotswold. More often a bushy bunch of wool projects straight out from the forehead. The Lincoln shears a heavy fleece because it is very long and dense and contains considerable yolk. The Lincoln and Cotswold resemble each other more closely than any other two breeds, and for this reason one must be familiar with the characteristics of the two breeds in order to distinguish between them.

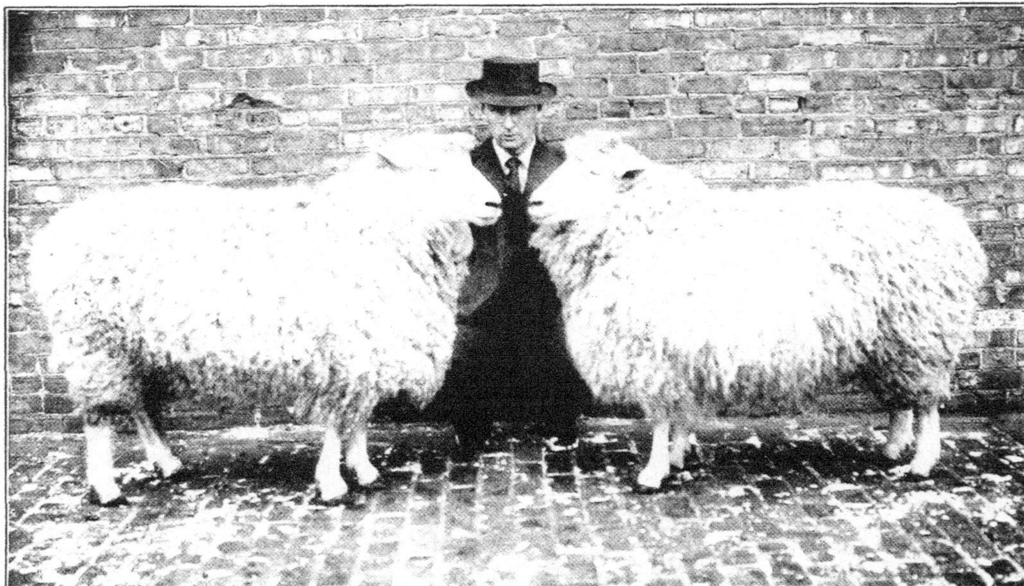

PLATE 92. First prize Lincoln ram and ewe lamb at the International, 1910; shown by Herbert Lee, Ontario, Canada.

STANDARD AND SCALE OF POINTS FOR LINCOLN SHEEP.

Constitution.—Body deep, back wide and straight; wide and full in the thigh; bright, large eyes; skin soft and of a pink color .	25
Size.—Matured rams not less than 250 pounds when in good condition. Matured ewes not less than 200 pounds	10
Appearance.—Good carriage and symmetry of form	10
Body.—Well proportioned, good bone and length; broad hind quarters; legs standing well apart; breast wide and deep . . .	15
Head.—Should be covered with wool to the ears; tuft on forehead; eyes expressive; ears fair length; dotted or mottled in color . .	10
Neck.—Medium length; good muscle; well set on body . . .	5
Legs.—Broad and set well apart; good shape; color white, but some black spots do not disqualify; wooled to the knees . . .	10
Fleece.—Of even length and quality over body; not less than eight inches long for one year's growth	10
Quality of Wool.—Rather fine, long wool; strong, lustrous fiber; no tendency to cot	5
Total	100

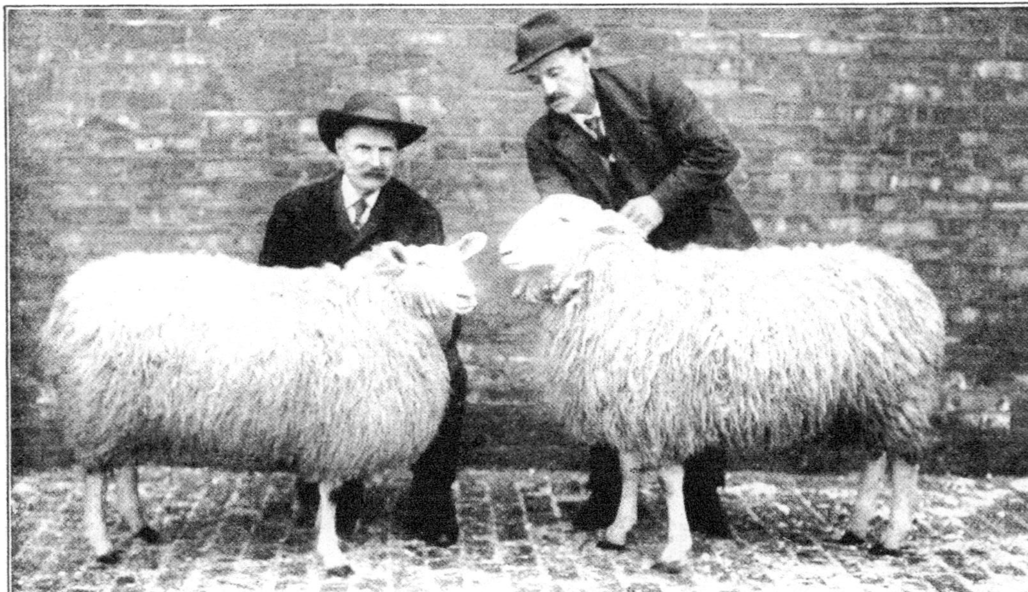

PLATE 93. First prize Leicester ram and ewe lamb at the International, 1910; shown by Whitlaw Bros., Ontario, Canada.

THE LEICESTER.

There is no difficulty in distinguishing this breed from any of the other long wools. The head is longer and somewhat narrower than the others. They have a tendency toward a Roman nose. This breed like the Cheviot and the Suffolk is absolutely bare of wool from the ears forward. The Leicester has a broad, well-fleshed back, but is generally shallower in body than the other long wools. That this breed has a more leggy appearance than the Cotswold or the Lincoln may be attributed to the fact that its wool is shorter, finer, and lighter over the body, especially on the belly. It is also finer in bone than the other two breeds. The fleece hangs in locks with small fine curls at the ends.

THE ROMNEY MARSH OR KENT.

This breed of sheep was probably first developed in Kent County, England, from stock which came originally from the Low Countries. A few small flocks have been imported to the United States.

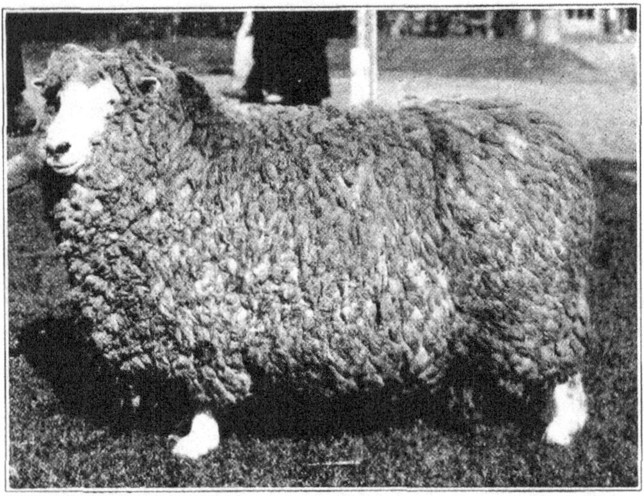

PLATE 94. First prize and champion Romney Marsh ram exhibited by Alfred Mathews, New Zealand, at the Panama Pacific Exposition, 1915. Courtesy of the American Sheep Breeder.

This breed has a strong masculine head, a short, strong neck, a wide deep chest, and is level along its back. It has a good spring of ribs, and is particularly full in the hindquarters. The fleece is of good length, but is not as long as that of the Lincoln. It is fairly dense and lustrous. It is desirable in this breed that the wool should open evenly, that is, there should be no cross fibers holding the locks together when the wool is parted.

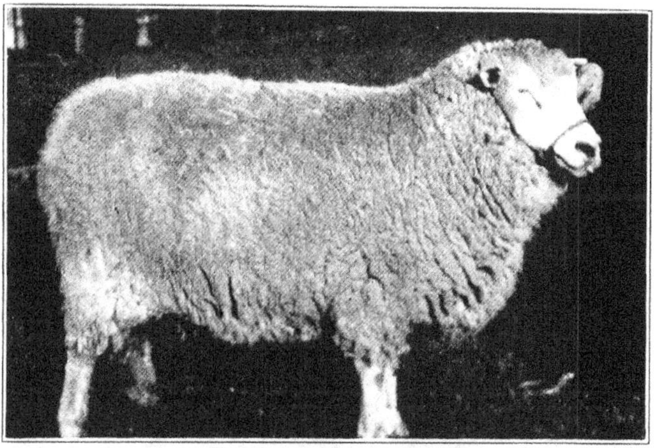

PLATE 95. First prize and champion Romney Marsh ewe exhibited by W. Riddel, Jr., of Oregon, at the Panama Pacific Exposition, 1915. Courtesy of the American Sheep Breeder.

This sheep has style, carries its head well up, and makes a good impression in general.

THE BLACK-FACED HIGHLAND.

This breed has its native home in Scotland where it thrives among the Scotch mountains. This is a horned sheep, the ram having much larger horns than the ewe. The color of the face varies from black, to black and white speckled, many having a big white star on the forehead. The legs are short, carrying a blocky, well-proportioned body. The wool on this breed is very long, hanging nearly to the ground when of a full year's growth. The fleece

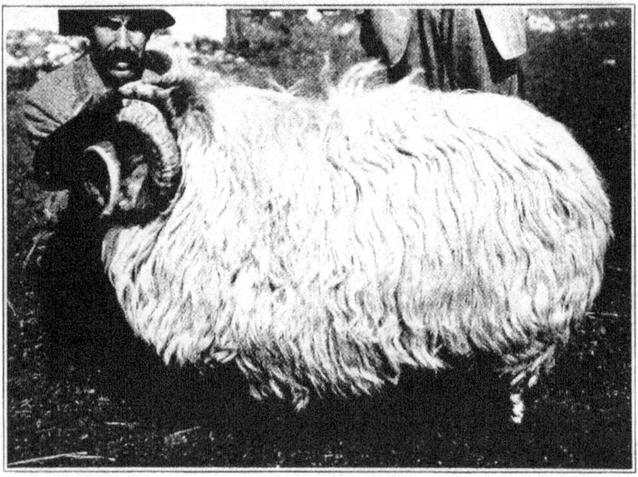

PLATE 96. First prize and champion Blackfaced Highland ram at the Scottish Shows, 1909. Courtesy of the American Sheep Breeder

is very coarse in fiber, however, and is generally used for the same purpose as that of the other long wool breeds; namely, the manufacture of the coarser kinds of woolen goods such as carpets or rugs. This breed has a very strong and robust constitution, which is necessary because of its native environment in the mountains. The Black-faced

Highland is often used for crossing with other breeds. When coming down the mountains, one trailing behind the other in a narrow path, a flock of this breed is a most beautiful sight.

THE CORRIEDALE.

The Corriedale sheep is a native of New Zealand. In the production and character of the breed as seen today, the breeders of that country mated Lincoln, Romney Marsh, and Leicester rams with Merino ewes. By careful selection of the rams used in crossing, the New Zealand breeder has produced a breed of sheep which not only shears a very good grade of wool, but also has a good mutton form. Today the Corriedale is a recognized breed and it is considered by the New Zealand breeders as nearly an ideal dual purpose sheep as can be found. Within the last few years small flocks of this breed have been imported to the United States. There were three exhibits of Corriedales at the Panama Pacific Exposition in 1915, and they were greatly admired by those who had never seen this sheep before. The accompanying illustration shows a Corriedale ram and ewe shown by King Bros. of Laramie, Wyoming.

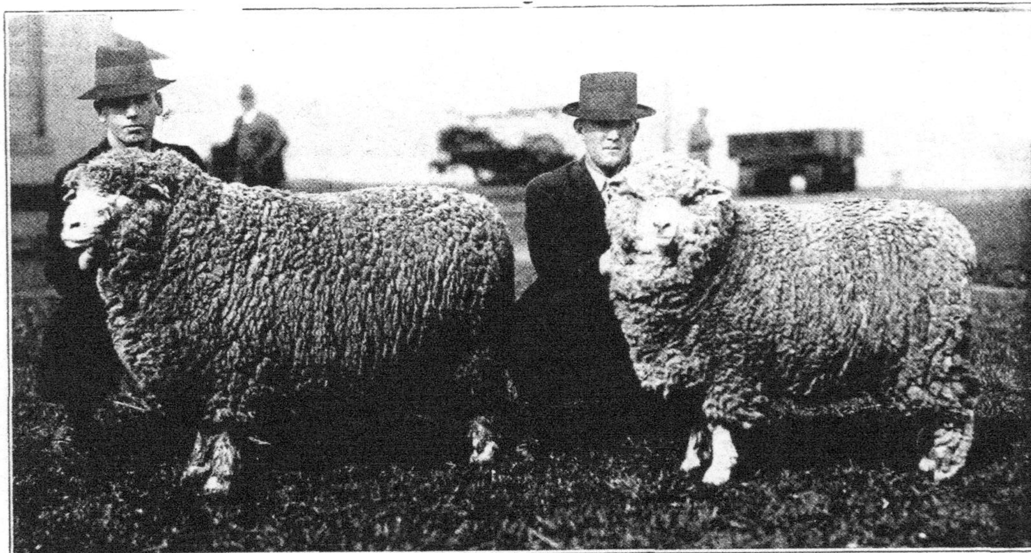

PLATE 97. Corriedale prize winning ram and ewe shown by King Bros., Laramie, Wyoming, at the Panama Pacific Exposition, 1915. Ram to the left, ewe right. Courtesy of the American Sheep Breeder.

OTHER LONG AND MEDIUM WOOLS.

There are a number of long and medium wool breeds which, so far as the writer knows, are not raised in America. At the great Royal Show in England other breeds raised in England and Scotland are seen which are unknown to the American shepherd. Among these breeds are found the Wensleydale; the Devon Long Wool; the Border Leicester, which is becoming very popular in New Zealand also; the South Devon, having characteristics very similar to the Devon Long Wool; the Herdwick; the Exmoor; the Ryeland, which in the writer's opinion is a very useful breed and undoubtedly would make a good cross on common western range ewes; the Roscommon; the Dartmoor, which is especially adapted to poor, hilly country; the Kerry Hill, and the Welsh breed. It is surprising how many different breeds of the long and medium wools are raised in Great Britain. There every flockowner carefully selects a breed suitable to the laying of his land and other conditions. As these men are thoroughly familiar with sheep husbandry, they have, as a rule, great success with their chosen breed.

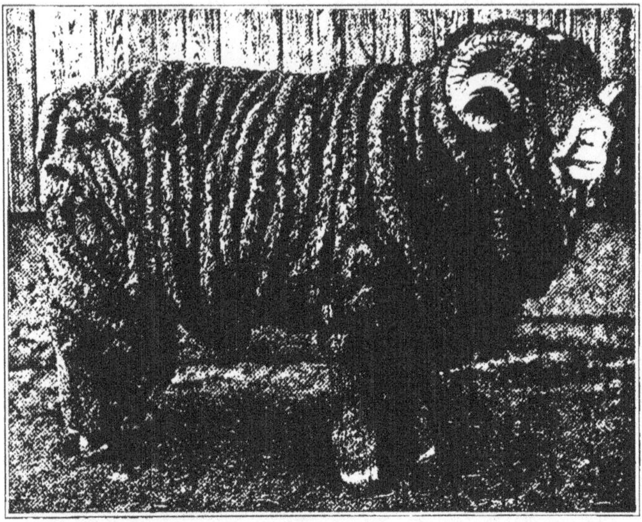

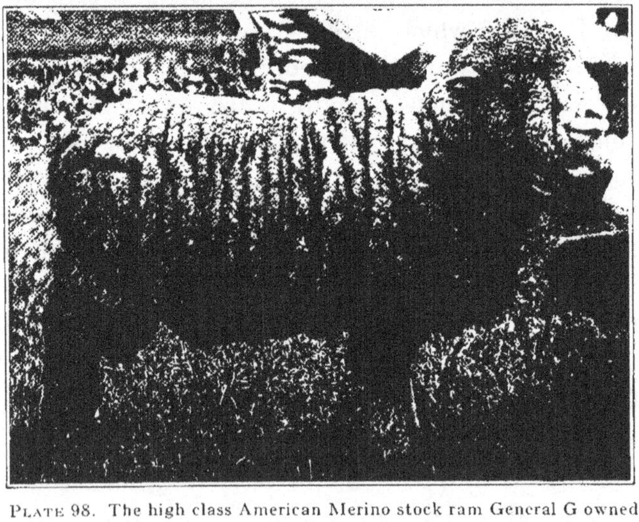

PLATE 98. The high class American Merino stock ram General G owned by W. M. Staley, Marysville, O, is shown above; a prize winning ewe, below. Courtesy American Sheep Breeder.

THE AMERICAN MERINO.

This breed originates from Spain, and as nearly as can be ascertained the first importation into this country was made in 1801. It is primarily a wool sheep, the wool being of the finest quality and containing a large amount of yolk. The fleece is so dense that it sheds water, which adds greatly to the sheep's extreme hardiness. The whole body from the nose down to the hocks is wrinkled. A heavy shearing is thus made possible by the many extra folds, the density of the wool and the great amount of yolk. Rams of this breed in one year's growth have produced fleeces from thirty-five to forty pounds. Wool covers this sheep from the nose to the feet. The color of the face, legs and ears is white. The rams have horns. In judging this breed at fairs, the quality and quantity of wool is the chief consideration. Only sufficient constitution and stamina are required to secure vigor. At the present time we do not find the American Merino exhibited at all of the state and county fairs.

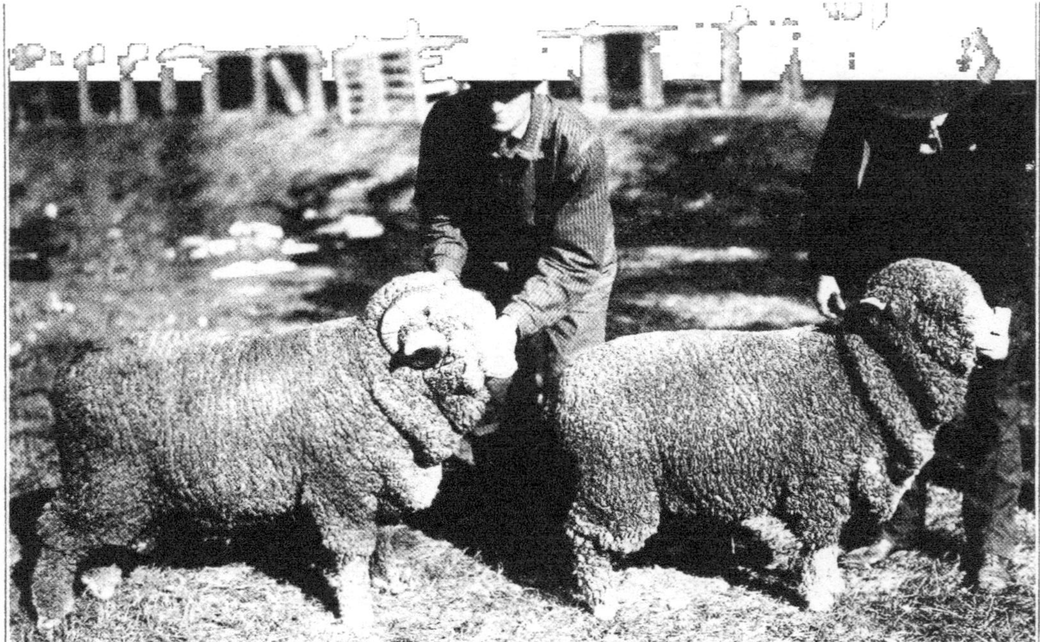

Plate 99. A very typical pair of Delaine Merinos. Ram to the left, ewe to the right. Courtesy American Sheep Breeder.

THE DELAINE MERINO.

The Delaine Merino has the same color of face and legs as the American. This breed differs from the first mentioned in general appearance, as it has not nearly so many wrinkles, having them only around its neck and breast, and some about the tail head. The fleece is generally not quite so dense, but a little longer and likewise of very good quality. Its form is usually better than that of the American, as it has a broader back and hindquarters. This breed is only considered as a wool sheep, but its appearance is more pleasing to the eye than that of the American.

The American and Delaine Merinos when shown together are often grouped into three types; A, B, and C. The A class has wrinkles all over the body; the B has wrinkles only around the neck and breast; while the C type is practically a smooth bodied sheep, having but one fold or wrinkle following the throat to the brisket where it joins another small semicircular fold.

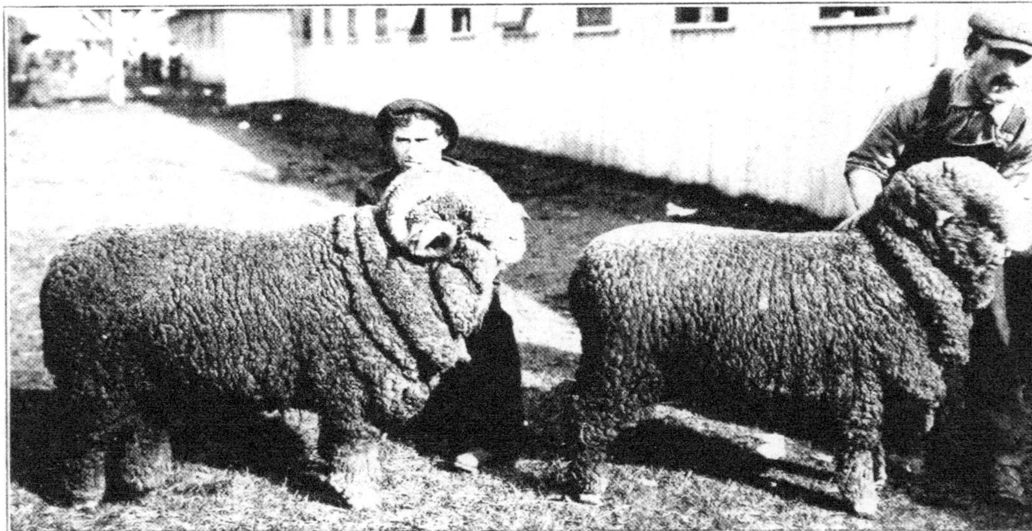

PLATE 100. Champion Rambouillet ram and ewe state fairs 1911. Ram on the left, ewe on the right. Shown by King Bros., Laramie, Wyo. Courtesy American Sheep Breeder.

THE RAMBOUILLET.

The Rambouillet is the largest and biggest framed of all the fine wool sheep. In this breed attention is paid not only to wool but to mutton as well. This sheep, which originated in France, has been so much improved in mutton form by careful breeding that it now compares fairly well with other mutton breeds. Breeders rate it as a dual purpose sheep, wool and mutton combined, and expect the judges at fairs in making the awards to allow fifty per cent for wool and type, and fifty per cent for mutton form.

The color of the face and legs is white, and the wool usually extends, like that of the Shropshire, from nose to toes. The fleece is dense, and of good quality, having perhaps less yolk than the other Merinos. They vary some in wrinkledness; some have larger folds on the neck and breast than others; and there is also some variation in the length and density of the wool. At the recent shows, two classes of Rambouillet sheep have been made, the B and the C types. The fine wool breeds must be given the credit of being the hardiest of all the breeds.

GRADES OF SHEEP ON OUR AMERICAN MARKETS.

The sheep market in America is divided into many different classes and grades. The wealthier consumers of mutton and lamb wish to get the choicest kind, regardless of the price, and this forces the firms to grade the live consignments into so many grades. This is in the favor of the producer. The one who has a choice lot of sheep or lambs is entitled to a higher price than the one who brings unfinished stuff to market, because he saved his feed, or perhaps did not have any. The breeding of the sheep which come to market makes a marked difference also. Sheep or lambs well bred, possessing a good mutton form, and furnishing many high price cuts, put on meat easily at a smaller cost and bring the highest prices. Today, the producer and shipper receive the price on the market according to the rating of their offerings. A lot which can be rated as prime or choice is much in favor, and a premium is paid for such a class. In all cases sheep do not bring as high prices as lambs. From all the sheep annually sent to market for slaughter about 75 per cent are lambs. Since buyers at the markets are always searching for the best and well finished classes of all grades, the breeder and feeder should aim to fulfill their requirements.

They are graded in the following manner:

MUTTON SHEEP (Mostly Westerns).

Lambs	Prime—handy weight from 70–80 lbs. Choice—weight from 75–85 lbs. Good. Medium. Common or Culls.
Yearlings	Prime—handy weight from 90–95 lbs. Choice—weight from 100–110 lbs. Good. Medium.
Wethers	Prime—handy weight from 105–110 lbs. Choice—weight from 110–125 lbs. Good. Common.
Ewes	Prime—handy weight from 90–95 lbs. Choice—weight from 95–110 lbs. Good. Medium. Common or Culls.
Bucks and Stags	Choice—weight from 150–185 lbs. Good. Common.

FEEDER CLASSES (Mostly Westerns).

Lambs	Choice— Good form and condition weighing from 55–60 lbs. Good— Fair condition weighing from 60–65 lbs. Common— In thin condition.
Yearlings	Choice— Good form and quality weighing from 85–90 lbs. Good— Fair in form and condition weighing 80–85 lbs. Common— Thin in condition and fair in form.

Wethers	Choice— Good quality and condition weighing 95–100 lbs. Good— Fair in quality and condition weighing 90–95 lbs. Common— Poor in flesh.
Ewes (*Westerns*)	Choice— Good condition and form (young) weighing 85–95 lbs. Good— Fair condition and form (young) weighing 80–90 lbs. Common— Thin (old).

BREEDING CLASSES.

Ewes	Choice— Young 2–3 years old. Good— 3–4 years old. Common— 5 years old.

Hot-House lambs for Christmas or Easter trade.
Fancy selected—weighing from 42–45 lbs.
Choice—weighing from 45–50 lbs.

INDEX

Made in the USA
Monee, IL
13 September 2026

62976739R00204